Mrs. Charlie

THE OTHER MAYO

A BIOGRAPHY

by

Judith Hartzell

Credits:
Written by Judith Hartzell
Design and Layout - Suzanne J. Curtis
Photo Contributors - Prudence Mayo Fox,
Dr. John Hartzell,
Mayo Kooiman, Penelope Mayo Lord
Charles Mayo Rankin, Edith Rankin Redden, and
Olmsted County Historical Society.
Also by permission of
The Mayo Foundation - Rochester, Minnesota,
Dorothy Angell Rutherford, and Random House, Inc.
Printing: Sentinel Printing Company, Saint Cloud, MN

ISBN 0-9703569-0-0 Price $16.95

Published By
Arvi Books, Inc. • 12 Sawgrass Court • Greenville, SC • 29609

Second Edition, 2015
www.judithhartzell.com

THIS BOOK IS DEDICATED TO PATIENTS AT THE MAYO CLINIC,
SO THAT THEY MAY KNOW SOME OF THE FOUNDING MAYO FAMILY'S
QUALITIES OF HEART AND SOUL

PREFACE

The life of Edith Graham Mayo is unlike many biographies written at the twentieth century's close, even though she was a twentieth century woman. Her character was formed in a pioneer Minnesota family — she benefited from the toughness, the sturdy faith, the neighborliness, and the strong hope for a bright and promising future which animates the pioneer. She was not confused, complex, or corrupted, like many late twentieth century characters.

I believe the quiet coherence of Edith Mayo's life can be an inspiration to us who came later. She was passionately devoted to healing the sick. Her marriage to Dr. Charles Horace Mayo delighted her not only because he was a lovable and entertaining man, but also because she could exercise her devotion to healing through all her efforts to encourage him and his brother in their work establishing the Mayo Clinic. And when tragedy struck her children, or any whom she loved, she could still see, in the great work done at the Clinic, her life fulfilling its purpose.

THANKS TO MANY WHO HELPED ME

This book has been a family work. It began because of a seed of curiosity planted in me by Esther Mayo Hartzell, who responded to my query, "What was your mother like?" with a quick, positive assertion: "My mother was a saint!" This puzzled me, coming from a woman who was not especially religious.

In the autumn of 1998, my husband, Thomas Mayo Hartzell, sent letters to all his cousins who might remember Edith Graham Mayo, asking for their recollections; she has 18 grandchildren still living. Mayo Kooiman quickly responded. She had just come into possession of a computer with e-mail capabilities, and it was a toy she enjoyed using. In addition, Granny had been a blessing in her young life, and Mayo was glad to recreate those years. She has a poetic soul. Tom and I eagerly collected the stories she sent us from October, '98, through June, '99. By then I had written a first draft of Edith's story. I sent it to some other cousins, hoping to provoke them to remember and write, and they did. We have had helpful collaboration in the text from Edith Mayo Rankin's children and granddaughter — Fred Rankin, Jr., his daughter Karin Rankin Sisk, Edith Rankin Redden, and Charles Mayo Rankin; from Dr. Chuck Mayo's children — especially Mildred ("Muff") Mayo, but also Dr. Charles H. Mayo II, Ned Mayo, Maria Mayo Donovan and her husband, Bernard Donovan; from Louise Mayo Trenholm's children — besides Mayo Kooiman, George and Lee Elwinger; and from Esther Mayo Hartzell's son Dr. John Mayo Hartzell. Also, Louise's daughter Penelope Lord has very graciously sent us many papers, photos, and even a VCR tape from her extensive collection of Mayo memorabilia, and Penny's twin sister Prudence Fox has sent some beautiful original photographs for me to use in the book. Edith Redden and Charles Rankin sent family photographs too, and Mayo Kooiman entrusted me with a sheaf of precious photos. My husband has been counseling and editing to help me from the start, and my son, Andy Hartzell, and good friends Sally Berk and Judy Stevens gave me valuable editorial advice. Without these people, this book would not have happened. Any mistakes in it, however, are my responsibility alone.

I want to thank the Olmsted County Historical Society too and its staff, especially Marilyn Hensley, Sherry Sweetman, and Barbara Dahlin, who helped me sort through their extensive collection of Mayo letters and photos. David Pennington of the O.C.H.S. board of directors assisted me in finding information and also kindly read the manuscript and offered editorial counsel. Dr. Carolyn Stickney Beck and Nicole Babcock were helpful with material in the Mayo Clinic archives. I gained valuable insight into Edith's and Hattie Mayo's characters from my interviews with Brunhilde Brunholzl, Dr. H. Frederic Helmholz, Jr., and Waltman Walters.

TABLE OF CONTENTS

GENEALOGY

Joseph Graham (1822-1914)	William Worrall Mayo (1819-1911)	Charles Horace Mayo (1865-1939)
&	&	&
Jane Twentyman (1828-1896)	Louise Abigail Wright (1825-1915)	Edith Maria Graham (1867-1943)

Mary Graham	(1847-1926)	Horace Mayo	(1851-1852)	Margaret Mayo	(1895-1895)
William Beck Graham	(1848-1940)	Gertrude Mayo	(1853-1938)	Dorothy Mayo	(1897-1960)
Thomas Graham	(1850-1936)	Phoebe Mayo	(1856-1885)	Charles William Mayo	(1898-1968)
John Graham	(1852-1869)	Sarah Mayo	(1859-1860)	Edith Mayo	(1900-1982)
Manfred Graham	(1854-1933)	William James Mayo	(1861-1939)	Joseph Graham Mayo	(1902-1936)
Christopher Graham	(1856-1952)	Charles Horace Mayo	(1865-1939)	Louise Mayo	(1905-1993)
Joseph Graham, Jr.	(1858-1949)			Rachel Mayo	(1908-1910)
Dinah Graham	(1860-1949)			Esther Mayo	(1909-1971)
Margaret Graham	(1862-1927)			Marilynn "Sally" Mayo	(1920-1984)
Frank Graham	(1864-1930)				
Edith Maria Graham	(1867-1943)				
Arthur Graham	(1869-1912)				
Jennie Graham	(1872-1897)				

The Five children of Edith and Dr. Charlie who had children

Charles William Mayo (Chuck) (1898-1968) & Alice Varney Plank (1907-1967)	Edith Mayo (1900-1982) & Fred W. Rankin (1886-1954)	Joseph Graham Mayo (1902-1936) & Ruth Rakowsky (1908-1942)	Louise Mayo (1905-1993) & George Trenholm (1902-1949)	Esther Mayo (1909-1971) & John B. Hartzell (1899-1970)
Mildred "Muff" Mayo (1928-2009)	Fred W. Rankin, Jr. (1924-2013)	David Graham Mayo (1930-1958)	George Mayo Trenholm (1929-2003)	John Mayo Hartzell (1931-)
Charles Horace Mayo II (1930-)	Edith "Missey" Graham Rankin (1926-)	William James Mayo II (1933-)	Mayo Trenholm (1930-2002)	Thomas Mayo Hartzell (1935)
Edward "Ned" Mayo (1931-)	Charles Mayo "Bo" Rankin (1927-)		Christopher Graham "Kit" Trenholm (1932-2014)	Ann Mayo Hartzell (1937-)
Joseph Graham Mayo II (1933-)	Thomas Rankin (1928-1985)		Robin Trenholm (1933-1933)	
Edith Maria Mayo (1937-)			Penelope Mayo Trenholm (1935-) & her twin sister, Prudence Mayo Trenholm (1935-2014)	
Alexander Mayo (1942-)				

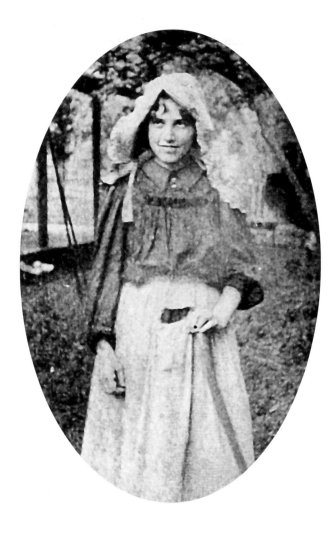

Edith Graham at about twelve,
taken at Grahamholm Farm

*Photo courtesy of Olmsted County Historical Society
and by permission of Dorothy Angell Rutherford*

Chapter 1

EARLY LIFE: PIONEERS IN MINNESOTA

"One day in February, when the weather was cold, the snow drifts deep, and the sky hung low and dark, Jane Twentyman Graham said to her son Christopher, 'You must go out and cut large chunks of snow. I have a great deal of laundry to do today, and it is important that I have plenty of hot water. Get along with you! Hurry, for it is almost lunch time.'"

So begins the story of Edith Maria Graham's birth on a winter's day in Minnesota, as told by her granddaughter Mayo Kooiman (hereafter referred to as "Mayo"). Kit Graham went outside, grumpy and complaining. Ten years old, he had other plans for that late morning. But at his mother's urging, he sawed big chunks of snow, looking around to find the cleanest. When he brought them inside, his mother quickly placed the snowchunks in a large pan on the stove. After four or five trips, the boy stood by the stove, watching the snow melt. His mother told him to bring in more wood and then go off and do something else.

"Lo and behold, not long after, his sweetest of all friends, Edith, had been born. He wrote his sister a letter on her sixtieth birthday, 'Had I known of your pending birth, I would have found even cleaner snow!'

"'My precious lady,' he said, 'you actually allowed me to be born that day. Nothing so important has ever made me so delighted in living. You surrounded my heart and have kept me thinking, challenged and solid all my life. You were the greatest gift, and what outshines even that – you have constantly and softly touched everyone I know. As I wish you happy birthday today, I can see you as a wee baby, just as if it were yesterday. Of course, you know this – I tell you every year.'" (This is from a letter Dr. Graham wrote Edith Mayo February 12, 1927.)

EDITH MARIA GRAHAM was born into two life-long passions – enjoying a large, close-knit family and healing the sick. From the moment she opened her eyes, on Tuesday, February 12, 1867, she was surrounded by a big, noisy, busy, loving family. Her parents, Jane Twentyman Graham and Joseph Graham, reared thirteen children, of whom Edith was the eleventh. She probably didn't remember her older brother John very well; he died at the age of seventeen when she was only two and a half. But the others thrived.

Alongside family life, Edith was introduced to nursing from her earliest years. She watched her mother care for all the children when they were sick, of course, as well as care for two babies who came after her, Arthur and Jennie. But Jane Graham's talent for nursing didn't stop with her own brood. She wanted to serve in the wider community, and so "she nursed all who needed her, without material gain" according to Clark Nelson, historian for the Mayo Clinic (in *Mayo Roots*).

Her special interest was in being a mid-wife. Mrs. Graham delivered 243 babies over the years, without any physician's help and without losing any mothers or children. This record was equaled by few doctors of her day. With such a mother as an example, both Edith and her older sister Dinah grew up to be nurses.

Edith learned more than compassion for the sick from her home life. Both parents taught her courage, stubbornness, and faith. These traits had enabled Joseph and Jane Graham to move from their farm home near Truxton, New York, to Minnesota Territory in May and June, 1856. They had joined a surge of immigrants to this land which the U.S. government had bought from Dakota Indians in July, 1851. In 1854 30,000 Americans of European descent lived in Minnesota Territory; three years later, 150,000 had settled there, eight of them Grahams. Jane had been only 17 when she married Joseph. When she was 28, she traveled to her new home beside her husband more than 1,000 miles in a covered wagon, together with their six children, the youngest at the start of their journey only a baby of eight weeks. Sioux Indians and some Winnebago still lived in southeast Minnesota when the Grahams arrived. According to a descendant of early settlers, "Even as late as 1856 the Indian still ruled the prairies and the stillness of the forests." But before Edith was born, all the Indians had moved on.

The Grahams were farmers, who traveled west looking for cheap and fertile land. This they found five miles northwest of what is now Rochester, in Kalmar Township, Olmsted County, where the going price of land in 1856 was $1.25 an acre. Joseph and Jane appear to have chosen their farm site wisely. The soil was rich, and two streams, forks of Cascade Creek, watered it.

At first, the Grahams raised Irish potatoes and other subsistence crops, managing to survive only with great effort in their new home, which they named "Grahamholm." In keeping with their Scottish and English heritage, they instilled in their children the virtues of thrift and hard, practical labor. As a young girl, Edith was responsible for milking the cows each morning and evening. At one point, she had had enough. Instead of rejoicing over the birth of a new heifer, she wept, knowing it would grow up soon, and there would be one more cow for her to milk.

At Christmastime, the Graham children prayed for small gifts in their stockings, but sometimes found only apples. They ran barefoot inside and out all spring, summer, and autumn. Shoes were too expensive to wear, except for the time of snows and ice. When the girls were old enough, Jane Graham taught each to do careful needlework in tiny hand-made stitches, creating quilts and clothing. One quilt, which Edith made when she was sixteen, was from sheets dyed dusty blue and cut into dark crescent moons and stars, sewn against a white background. Because the family was frugal, Edith's mother gave her worn sheets to work with, not new ones, which would have been used by wealthier girls.

Edith was a natural athlete and loved riding horses. At that time, girls and women were expected to ride sidesaddle. But the Grahams couldn't afford a saddle for their little daughter, much less a sidesaddle, so she rode bareback. She later told her granddaughter Mildred "Muff" Mayo (hereafter referred to as "Muff") about her riding: "I would always sit on a horse astride and make him go fast," she said, "like the wind over the prairies, except when passing a farm. Then I would throw my leg over, so as not to be seen astride by the folk. But the moment the horse and I were by, I'd throw my leg back over and away we'd be!"

Edith's parents were determined to educate their children the best they could. Fortunately, Grahamholm was located near Kalmar Township District School Number 24, which was erected by a school-raising party of local parents the same year Jane and Joseph Graham arrived in Minnesota. Their children could easily walk the mile and three-quarters to school along the road, or they could follow a shorter route along the creekbed which ran diagonally through their father's property, from near the house to school. Edith probably attended this school from first through eighth grade.

During the years Edith was a student, the public schools of Olmsted County were unusually good. Sanford Niles improved them during his 11 year tenure as Olmsted County Superintendent of Schools. He began his work in 1865, two years before Edith was born. During his first year superintending, he visited all 77 schools in the county and, according to Harriet Hodgson, author of *Rochester, City of the Prairie*, "was horrified to discover that 56 had no outhouses and 11 no blackboards." These defects were corrected long before Edith arrived at School Number 24.

Niles cared not only for buildings, but also textbooks and teachers. In fact, he became one of the most famous men in Olmsted County at that time because he wrote textbooks that sold throughout the United States, such as *History of the United States* and *Advanced Geography*. He also wrote the first curriculum for students in Minnesota and set up programs to both train and test teachers in nine areas: reading, writing, grammar, spelling, geography, United States history, civics, hygiene and math.

His ideas on education were advanced. Edith benefited from his belief that students should be constant observers, self-reliant and creative. Teachers were not to teach in the commonly accepted way, by rote. No, said Niles, reading was to be taught in an "easy, natural manner, similar to daily conversation," and lessons were in themes or topics which would pique a child's interest. Because of Niles' diligence, Edith's education at the little township school was superior.

However, her primary teachers were always her

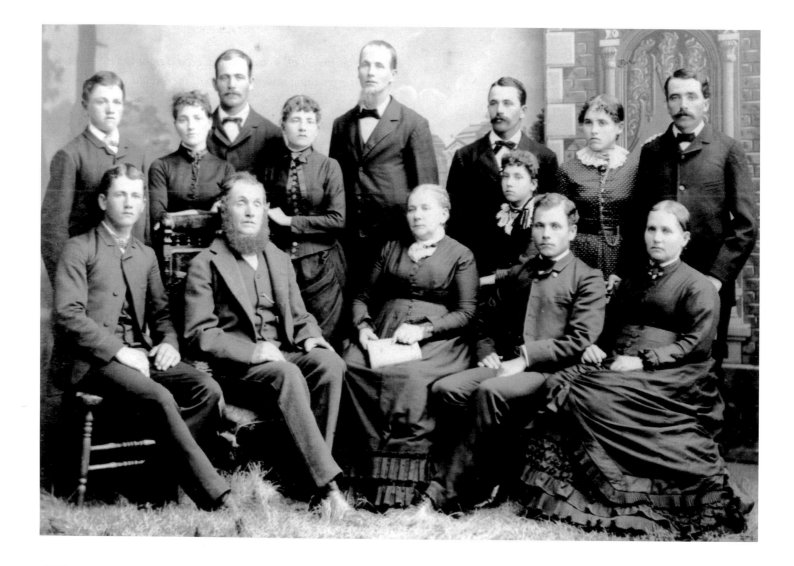

The Joseph Graham/Jane Twentyman Graham Family in 1895.
Standing, left to right: Arthur Graham, Dinah Graham (Mrs. Mark Olin), Joseph Graham, Jr., Margaret Graham (Mrs. William Twentyman), William Beck Graham, Thomas Graham, Edith Graham (Mrs. Charles H. Mayo), and Manfred Graham.
Seated, left to right: Frank Graham, Joseph Graham, Sr., Jane Twentyman Graham, Jennie Graham (Mrs. Walter Williams), Christopher Graham and Mary Graham (Mrs. William Robert Waldron)

Photo courtesy of Olmsted County Historical Society

parents. Years later, her brother Kit described their early influence: "Our... scanty young experience maybe did no harm. We had our visions, dreams, hopes – and all were magnified because our real gifts...were meagre. Yet, Mother gave us much of her experience of England and New York that enlivened our passing days, and led us decently on, not down....When I think of [England], and its memories that Mother first gave us, and [which] Father intensified…,well, it just smells of Heaven, if smells, beauty and Heaven are one....Father gave us much more than our younger days would admit. We got no bad from him, so it looks at this distance. Honesty he taught by word and deed – clearly more so than most men."

Judging from an essay Edith composed just before her fourteenth birthday, she had plenty of faith in the abilities of intelligent women like her mother, her sisters, and herself. She entitled the essay

"Women's Rights"

"Now first of all women have as good a right to vote as men. And if every thing was as it should be they would vote....The idea of women not knowing enough to hold office, where you see one smart man you see a dozen smart women. And to hear a man say a woman don't [sic] know enough to hold office, when he is scarcely more than a fool himself is ridiculous. And I say that a woman who will listen to it don't [sic] know her own mind but ought to learn it.

"I think a woman has as good a right to be President as a man and would raise Congress right along if she could be Secretary of State or something of this kind. And I think it is just awful the way they have to make [women] scrub, milk, dig holes, etc. when they were born to something higher. But No, their brothers must have the education, he must not work, he must be king if possible. He is a boy.

"Yes, that is the way, but it won't be [for] long if I can help it. Follow my example, girls, and we will soon vote, and hold office, be President, and serve in Congress."

She signs the essay *"E.M.G., Esquire."*
(Not enough girls followed Edith's example; the state of Minnesota didn't grant women the right to vote until 1919, when she was 52.)

After completing her public school education, Edith taught in Olmsted County. But by the time she was twenty, she and Dinah had convinced themselves

Edith as a young woman, about eighteen years old

Photo courtesy of Mayo Kooiman

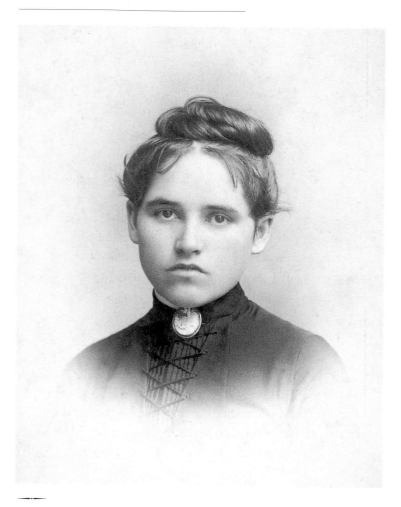

to follow their mother's path. They and two friends, who were also sisters, applied to be nursing students at Women's Hospital in Chicago, the nearest place which offered professional training. Edith asked the superintendent of public schools in Olmsted County, J. H. Chapman, Jr., to write a recommendation for her, and he was happy to oblige. Here is his assessment of Edith's abilities in 1887: "I take pleasure in stating that I have been acquainted with Miss Edith Graham for some time and know her to be a young lady of unquestionable character, a good scholar and one who has proven herself to be a very successful teacher. Miss Graham is faithful and industrious in whatever work she undertakes."

Undergirding Edith's life from childhood through old age was an unquestioned faith in God. As a girl, Edith wrote this poem:

> *"When I am weary and tired*
> *And in need of love,*
> *I look to the dark sky*
> *And know God is above.*
> *The moon gives a glow*
> *And the stars give new lease.*
> *It makes me calm*
> *And grants me great peace*
> *And grants me great peace."*

Chapter 2

Nursing and Putting People to Sleep

It was a glad day for the Graham family when Edith graduated from Chicago Women's Hospital's nursing program on April 7, 1889. To become a nurse in those days meant accepting duties of the most menial servant, hoping to perform them with the love of a saint. At least, that was Edith's idea of nursing, as she had seen it demonstrated in her mother's life. The family originally expected a double celebration, Edith and Dinah too. But Dinah contracted pneumonia in Chicago and had to drop out of the program; when she recovered, she returned to nursing school and graduated a year after Edith, in 1890.

At 22, Edith was short – five feet two and one-half inches – , small of person and vivacious, with brown hair and big brown eyes. She was assigned by Women's Hospital as nurse to a Chicago doctor, but when she reported for duty, he fired her on the spot. "Too young and too beautiful," he explained. So Edith returned home to Rochester, looking for work.

Dr. William Worrall Mayo was not a man to allow a woman's beauty to obscure her professional qualifications. His practice in Rochester was prospering. Patients came to him from 40 miles away in all directions, and some from as far as Iowa and South Dakota. He and his two sons, Dr. William James Mayo and Dr. Charles Horace Mayo, treated patients in their office and visited them in their homes, where they sometimes performed surgery. (Rochester, like most small towns, had no hospital.)

In the office, Dr. W.W. Mayo was often assisted by his wife, Louise. Slightly taller than he, Louise had energy, determination and intelligence quite equal to his. She had educated herself in medicine, botany and astronomy. Once, she doctored a patient with a dislocated shoulder when she passed the door of another Rochester doctor, and he called her in to help. Taking off her shoe, she placed her foot against the shoulder and put it right with a hefty pull. Louise's can-do attitude convinced her husband that women could do whatever they put their minds to.

Because Louise had many household duties, she could not handle all the nursing demands of her husband's growing practice. He needed a replacement. In Edith Graham, he thought he detected some of the intelligence and resourcefulness his wife possessed. When Dr. Mayo hired Edith, she became the first professionally trained nurse in Rochester.

Edith, from the beginning, displayed a determination to learn and a way of handling patients that endeared her to her employer. Her ability to ride horseback added to her value: when Dr. Mayo needed follow-up nursing for a country patient, he sent Edith on a horse.

Always, Dr. Mayo was patient and supportive with

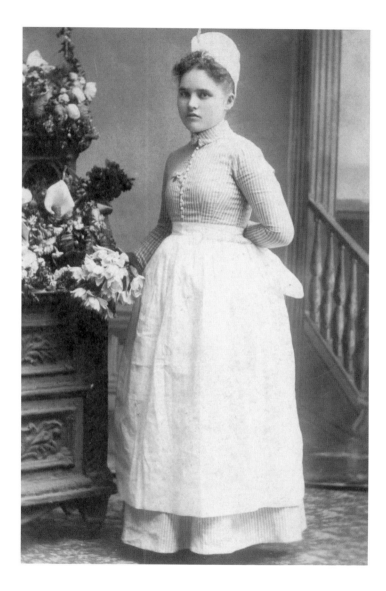

her, though with other people he was sometimes irascible and quick-tempered. According to her son Dr. Chuck Mayo, "Grandfather, uncharacteristically, adored her wholeheartedly."

He wasn't alone in feeling this way. "All her life, the young doctors at the Clinic were falling in love with her," Dr. Chuck said. She was "a radiant and truly beautiful woman…."

In addition to Edith, others in the Mayo practice were young in the spring of 1889, when she was hired. Dr. Will was 27 and Dr. Charlie 23; both appeared younger than their years. All three sometimes found their youthful looks to be drawbacks in treating patients. The brothers dubbed their early years of practice, "toe-in-the-door days." Often, when their father sent them to answer a call for "Dr. Mayo," they had to stick a toe into the partly-closed door and argue their right to be admitted, for the patient had called for, and insisted upon, the older Dr. Mayo, the one people called "the little doctor." (He was, by his own description, "small of stature, five feet four, thin of flesh, weighing 120 pounds, but wiry and active and capable of great endurance and fortitude." This is from a newspaper account he wrote when he was 36.)

If the little doctor's patients wanted to turn away Dr.

Will and Dr. Charlie, they were no happier when he trained 22-year-old Edith to be his anesthetist. At that time, anesthetics, usually chloroform, were administered by male interns. But the interns often became so interested in watching operations, they would forget to watch the patients. As a result, too many surgery patients died from chloroform poisoning. Disturbed by this problem, Dr. Mayo took a bold step. He believed an intelligent woman like Edith could learn to give chloroform better than these interns. So he taught her to watch the patient's blood pressure, pulse, reflexes, and dryness of the skin and eyes, and to adjust the chloroform dose accordingly. She soon became an expert. When patients saw how young Edith was, though, they were often nervous, so the little doctor stood beside her to reassure them until they fell asleep.

In the fall of 1889, Dr. Mayo united the Mayo medical practice with a hospital, and Edith's life immediately grew much busier. The idea for the hospital dated back to 1883, when a tornado struck Rochester, killing 31 people, injuring scores more, and damaging 172 homes. Mother Alfred Moes, director of the Sisters of St. Francis (a Catholic teaching order), and her nuns assisted Dr. Mayo and other town doctors in caring for the injured. For emergency hospitals, they used Rommel's Dance Hall

and every other building not in daily use.

After the crisis passed, Mother Alfred suggested to Dr. Mayo that together they build a permanent hospital. She was firm in her idea, telling him she had received a vision from the Lord directing her to establish a hospital with Dr. Mayo its director. It would become "world renowned for its medical arts," she said.

At first, Dr. Mayo was against the idea, believing the town to be too small and a hospital too costly. In those days, before the use of antiseptic agents in surgery, wounds commonly became infected. Smelly from putrefying flesh, and gloomy, city hospitals offered care inferior to home care. People considered hospitals in the same class as jails and asylums for the mentally ill – as places for people too poor to go anywhere else. Of the early days at St. Mary's Hospital, Edith told the biographer Helen Clapesattle, "We almost had to lock some of the first patients in their rooms; they were so sure they were going to die if they came" (quoted in *The Doctors Mayo*).

Dr. Mayo argued with Mother Alfred that a hospital would probably fail, since people who could pay for their care would stay home. Also, at 64, he thought he was too old to be involved. Mother Alfred disagreed, pointing out he had two sons who could help him. She persuaded the little doctor to back the hospital idea, organized the raising of funds, and purchased the property. Meanwhile, Dr. Mayo and

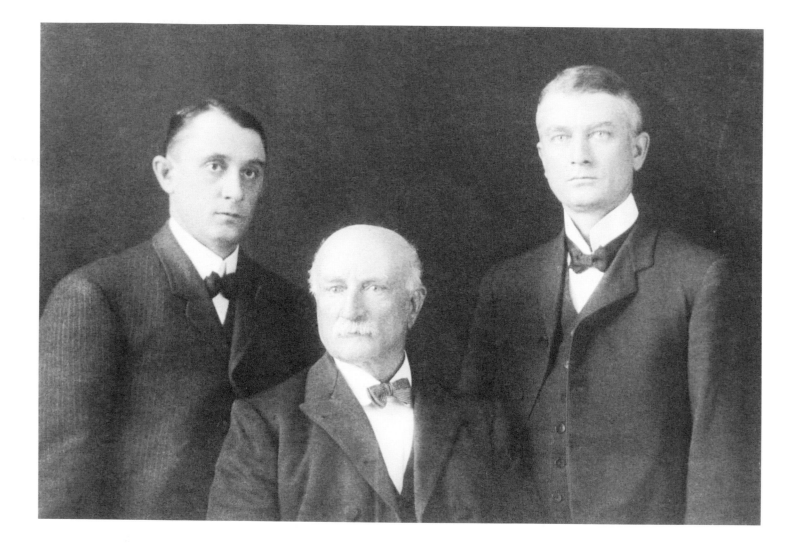

his sons gathered information on how to build an up-to-date facility. Construction began, and on September 30, 1889, St. Mary's Hospital opened with 45 beds. It was the first American hospital to use aseptic and antiseptic surgery methods from its beginning. Dr. Charlie performed the first operation, removing a cancer of the eye.

In the days to follow, Edith Graham's new task was to turn teaching nuns into nurses, and this was, at first, not easy. For instance, she had a problem with Sister Joseph. The first time Sister Joseph was asked to assist at examining a patient, she ran to a corner of the room and stood facing the wall, outraged and ashamed, because the patient, a man, was to be examined naked. She told Edith it was impossible for her to be a nurse; she planned to transfer back to teaching immediately. Edith not only convinced her to stay but also proved so persuasive that, less than three years later, Sister Joseph, now head of the hospital, became known as a person absolutely opposed to prudery, if it conflicted with good nursing.

For several weeks after the hospital opened, Edith conducted nursing classes for the nuns. Then she transferred most hospital nursing duties to them, so she could become the hospital anesthetist. On days when surgery was scheduled, she would come in early to make sure everything was ready. After administering the anesthetic, she nursed the patient throughout the day. In addition, she continued to serve as Dr. W. W. Mayo's nurse and secretary, writing his letters and sending out his bills.

Of the first 400 patients admitted to St. Mary's Hospital, only two died. This was a remarkable record. The credit was due to skillful surgery by all three Doctors Mayo; careful administration of anesthetics by Edith Graham and later her sister Dinah; and patient, prayerful, intelligent nursing by Edith, Dinah and the Sisters of St. Francis.

Dinah Graham joined the Mayo practice in the spring of 1890 as nurse for Dr. Will, anesthetist at St. Mary's, and bookkeeper in the Mayo office. The practice was expanding, and in February, 1892, Dr. Mayo added another partner besides his sons, Dr. Augustus W. Stinchfield, known as the best doctor in the Rochester area besides the Mayos. Then Dr. Mayo, 72, more or less retired, though his interest in the Mayo practice never ceased until his death on March 6, 1911 at the age of 91.

Edith's son Dr. Chuck later described his grandfather's evolving medical ideas as his "master plan," which grew into the first private group medical practice in America, the Mayo Clinic. "Father and

Uncle Will had something extra to offer [over other surgeons]: group medicine, with total teamwork. The Mayos had been raised to work together, pooling their skills and insights; when it came time to pick partners because of the pressure of the work, they selected [persons] with cooperative natures and a high degree of skill in areas which complemented their own." (A precept Will and Charlie learned from their father which, according to Clapesattle, they often repeated was "No man is big enough to be independent of others.")

Summing up the master plan, Dr. Chuck said, "This concept of interlocking talents and a mood of sharing, evolving as it did from Grandfather's zealous grooming of his sons, is the fundamental reason why the Mayo Clinic is so respected today. It had started with a strong, loyal family working together and it retained that clan spirit."

An important part of the group from the beginning was Edith Graham, who became part of the family, the other Mayo, as Dr. Charlie's wife.

⟶

Chapter 3

MARRIAGE TO DR. CHARLIE

Charlie was one of the first people in Rochester to buy a bicycle. Edith quickly learned to ride, and they began taking bicycle trips together about town and into the country. With a group of friends their own age, they enjoyed picnics and hayrides. In winter, since both were strong skaters, they skated together at ice-skating parties. As they continued to work closely together, each came to admire the other's skill and dedication to healing the sick, and friendship intensified into courtship.

Judging from some letters Charlie wrote in November, 1892, he fell in love with Edith during that winter, and once he was sure of his feelings, he quickly acted upon them. On November 22 Charlie wrote Edith a friendly, but hardly passionate, letter from Chicago, where he and his father had gone to observe surgeons, especially Dr. Nicholas Senn: "Every morning we get up at 4 and go out to see Senn work at St. Joseph's Hospital, then in the afternoon meet him again at 2 o'clock in the Presbyterian Hospital...."

It was a letter one might write to a nice nurse. However, he did end with a note that suggests she was teasing him a bit: "Let me know about the dance you would not invite me to go to. Yours truly, C.H. Mayo."

Four days later his letter was warmer. He had received a letter from her, and she was still teasing him. "You said nothing to satisfy our curiosity as to who took you to the dance. But it is just like the girls to tell just a little – enough to arouse curiosity and then quit," he chided gently.

Edith was now administering ether for the Drs. Mayo, and doing it better than the Chicago intern-anesthetists. Charlie suggested, "We shall have to give you a week off to let you come down here and show them how to give ether."

Then he signed as he did the earlier letter, adding three little words, "Love to all, Yours truly, C.H. Mayo."

Charlie proposed early in February, which is a big leap forward from these cautious letters, and Edith accepted. According to a story told by their granddaughter Muff, the engagement occurred shortly after a church supper at which a game was played during dessert. The baker had baked a ring into the cake, and whoever selected the cake piece with the ring was supposed to receive a big blessing. But they didn't find the ring that night, even though the girl in charge looked everywhere for it, even in Dr. Charlie's mouth. His merry eyes made her think he might be hiding it there.

And he was cleverly hiding it there. The next place it was seen was on Edith's finger – Charlie had impulsively used the play ring to propose to her that very night. He also gave her a book of poems by Ella Wheeler Wilcox, *An Erring Woman's Love*. Possibly all of this took place on her twenty-sixth birthday, February 12th.

When Edith conveyed the news of her engagement to her family, they were overjoyed. Her sister Jenny

Graham wrote from St. Paul on February 17,
"*My dear Edith:*

When we got home this noon, we were very much pleased to find a letter from you. We opened it never dreaming of the good news it contained. You can hardly imagine how pleased we are. And it is my prayer that you may be very very happy. Of course you will be, for he is so good and noble, and I know you are worthy of each other. Dear Edith, I can't express myself properly, but you will take the will for the deed. I have been perfectly happy the whole afternoon, because I know you are happy."

That same day Edith's niece Musetta Graham wrote:
"*Dearest Edith:*

Your letter and the sweet secret have been received, and although it was somewhat of a surprise, still it was the sweetest and most welcome surprise I ever had....You will always be happy. You couldn't be otherwise with so kind and noble a man to care for you, and you are worthy of everything. There is nothing good or beautiful of which you are not worthy....Edith, I am happy in your sweet, pure happiness....I can't express the true joy I feel for you on paper....Give my love to the one whom you love and who loves you, and say to him for me that he has made us all glad as no one else could have done.

Lovingly yours, Musie."

There is no record anywhere that anyone in the Graham family held a different opinion of the match, or that anyone ever changed from wholehearted endorsement of Charles Mayo as husband for their beloved Edith. On the contrary, many later letters tell of the family's gratitude for extremely kind deeds he did for them. He cared for them and their children in illness without charge; he promoted the careers of three of Edith's siblings, Dinah, Christopher, and William Beck Graham. Most of his kindnesses were quietly done and remain off record, but these examples show why he was a great favorite of the Graham family his entire life.

What kind of man was Charles Mayo to inspire his in-laws with such delight? He was a dynamo of energy and ideas. Already, he was a skilled doctor and surgeon, giving promise of becoming a great one. He was short – five feet five and a half inches – and strong, weighing 128 pounds. In appearance, he was dark-complected and good looking, with very dark brown hair and big, expressive brown eyes over-arched by thick, bushy eyebrows. He loved animals, children, plants and flowers, farming, and music. He had a genius for mechanical things, was full of fun and joie de vivre, and, most important to a bride, he loved her ardently.

Charlie had been born in Rochester in the Mayo house on Franklin Street July 19, 1865, the last of six children. At the time of his birth, his mother was going on 40 and his father was 46. His brother William was almost four years older than he. His two sisters were Gertrude, just turned twelve, and Phoebe, nine. Two other children, Horace and Sarah Frances, had already died. (Charlie's middle name, "Horace," was given him in memory of his deceased brother.)

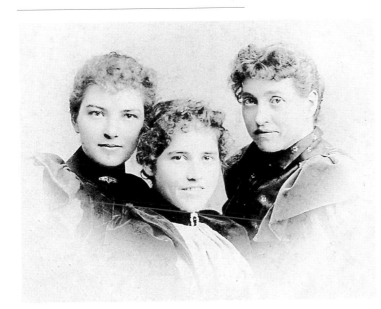

From the beginning, the father took charge of his sons' education. He had been on the board of education during the time Rochester Central Grade School, which both boys attended, was planned and built. When they had learned all they could there, he paid for them to go to the Niles School, a private high school in Rochester run by Sanford Niles after he was voted out of the superintendent's office. Here their preparation was unusually good. Afterwards, Dr. Mayo sent Will to the University of Michigan Medical School, after carefully checking out all the options, and, to gain a different perspective, he sent Charlie to Chicago Medical College, which was nominally tied to Northwestern University.

But the boys' chief teacher in medicine was always their father. The most important shaping force of the Mayo boys' childhood and youth, according to their biographer Clapesattle, "appears natural and inevitable: They helped their father in his work…, and so they were learning the practice of medicine almost from their cradle days." At first they cared for their father's horse while he was attending patients. Then, as a young teen, Will began to assist with surgeries while Charlie, still a child, stood by with strands of silk and linen for his father to use tying off blood vessels.

Once when Charlie was nine, the doctor acting as anesthetist became nauseated in the middle of a gruesome operation to remove an abdominal tumor from a woman and ran from the house. Charlie was summoned to help. As Dr. Charlie later told the story, "I stood on a box at the head of the table, dropping chloroform. When she stopped wiggling Father would tell me to stop, and when she started I would drop some more. I did fine."

Reflecting later on their lives as physicians, Dr. Will said, "To grow up in a doctor's family with a professional background of some generations will likely have, as it did with my brother and myself, that sort of influence which leads, not to conscious choice of medicine as a career, but rather to unconscious elimination of every other choice. Neither my brother nor I ever had an idea of being anything but a doctor."

Charlie's dedication to medicine was a powerful attraction for Edith, because she shared it. Her son said, "Mother was as consecrated to medicine as any Mayo." When Dr. Chuck began medical school years later, she wrote him a letter of encouragement, revealing how highly she valued the doctor's work. "Medicine," she wrote, is "the greatest profession in the world, not excepting the ministry....A doctor's calling is a sacred calling and only high-minded men should enter the ranks." When Edith agreed to become Dr. Charlie's wife, she set herself to support his work with every resource of intelligence, compassion, energy and understanding she possessed.

Edith married Charlie at 4:30 p.m. Wednesday, April 5, 1893, in the parlor of her parents' home at 801 South Genessee Street, Rochester, where they had moved from Grahamholm. The wedding was a happy occasion which the Rochester newspaper called "one of the neatest and at the same time one of the most quiet home weddings that has occurred in some time." Vases of cut flowers and lilies, as well as potted plants, decorated the parlor. Edith, according to the newspaper, "was extremely beautiful in a dress of cream silk crepe." It was trimmed at the high neckline and hem of its long, full skirt with ecru lace and had puffed three-quarter sleeves. The dress, now in the collection of Mayo memorabilia at Olmsted County Historical Society, to a modern eye looks very small.

Edith's dear friend and only bridesmaid, Alice Magaw, wore a cream crepe dress also, trimmed in Nile green. Dr. Charlie chose Edith's brother Dr. Kit Graham for his best man. (Charlie's brother was on a surgery inspection trip.) Concluding the ceremony, and preparing the way for "an elaborate supper," Daisy Berkman, Dr. Charlie's 15-year-old niece, played a spirited piano version of the wedding march. The newspaper writer concluded, "The happy couple deserve and will receive all of prosperity and connubial bliss that can fall to the lot of mortal."

What would be more natural to a man so steeped in medicine as Dr. Charlie than to take his bride on a tour of hospitals? It was their honeymoon trip. They left for New York City by train the evening of their wedding and spent five weeks in the East, followed by two weeks in Chicago, visiting surgical centers. Edith was pleased with the itinerary. Unlike other surgeons' wives, who liked to shop and visit the theater while their husbands inspected hospitals, Edith preferred operating rooms. She also enjoyed meeting Charlie's doctor friends, and they quickly became her friends as well.

After her wedding, Edith resigned as nurse in the Mayo practice, but she never ceased learning about surgery and nursing. She "had opinions on every subject under the sun, especially the Clinic, and she was capable of expressing herself with tact, but unmistakably...," according to her son. Edith always remained, in spirit, part of the practice. This was easy for her to do because she heard Clinic news from her husband and also from Alice Magaw, who was hired and trained as anesthetist at St. Mary's to replace Edith. She was the only anesthetist there until 1900. So effective was Alice in administering ether, she began writing papers on how to do it. In 1904 she gave a talk to the Minnesota Medical Society, telling of what she had learned from 11,000 patients whom she had anesthetized without a single death; an admiring Iowa doctor said she was able to "talk her patients to sleep." Alice became, in the early 1900's, the most famous member of the Mayo practice apart from Dr. Will and Dr. Charlie. She visited often in Edith's home.

Returning to Rochester from their wedding trip, Charlie and Edith moved right into "the yellow house" in Rochester on the corner of College and Dakota Streets, the home Dr. Will shared with his wife, the former Hattie May Damon. This arrangement seemed perfectly natural to the brothers; Charlie had lived there before his marriage also. The younger couple lived with the older for the following two years, while their own home, "the red house," was being built right next door.

Will and Hattie had been married eight and one-half years in the spring of 1893. Hattie, who was 29, had already given birth to three children, of whom only one, Carrie Louise, six, survived. Another baby, William, was destined to die while Edith and Charlie were still in the yellow house.

Hattie was quite different from Edith. Quiet and shy, she found conversing with visiting doctors difficult. But she was at ease with the wealthy and socially privileged families of Rochester; her father, Eleazer Damon, was a prosperous man, the only jeweler in Rochester and one of the city aldermen. Reared as an only child after her sister died as a baby, Hattie was, according to her grandson Waltman Walters, "regal....Just by being there, she ruled the room."

After graduating from the Niles School, Hattie completed a year at Carleton College, dropping out of the degree program to marry Dr. Will at age twenty. She was artistic, enjoyed painting, and worked enthusiastically with the St. Paul firm of Ellerbe & Rounds in designing the two beautiful homes which Dr. Will and Hattie built, lived in, and eventually donated to the Clinic – Mayo Foundation House and Damon House. She was also active in the American Organization of University Women and the League of Women Voters.

Hattie treated her husband more formally and with more diffidence than Edith treated Charlie. For instance, Hattie "would never have dreamed of disagreeing with [Dr. Will] or failing to follow his wishes, or of offering the slightest opinion on affairs at the Clinic, which she considered to be none of her business," according to Dr. Chuck. Nevertheless, despite their differences, the two women liked, respected and enjoyed one another; they were lifelong friends.

In some circles, the disparity between the wives'

fathers' social positions – poor farmer rearing thirteen children, rich jeweler rearing one girl – might have led to a social gulf between them. But the Mayos – in their families as in their medical practice – were thorough meritocrats. Whoever was able and of good character was attractive as a friend or colleague of the Doctors Mayo. Similarly, Edith and Hattie each recognized the other's worth; they always associated as equals.

Both wives honored their husbands' friendship almost without reservation. The respect and love the brothers shared was legendary. Clapesattle said, "It is hard to believe but undeniably true that the two men had only one pocketbook, one bank account, between them." Whatever either brother earned went into this bank account; each wrote checks on the account for whatever he needed – entertainment, travel, clothes, houses, cars, everything – without accounting to the other. All the checks read simply, "Drs. Mayo." At the end of the year, the monies left over they divided equally. Such was the trust between them.

Dr. William D. Haggard, a surgeon from Nashville, Tennessee, and a friend of both brothers, wrote Dr. Will much later, "Your great success was not as surgeons. It was as brothers. There has never been anything like it."

Not surprisingly, neither Hattie nor Edith complained when Charlie built, next door, an almost exact duplicate of Will's house – including a fully equipped game room. The women enjoyed watching their husbands rock back and forth together in an unusual piece of furniture which Charlie kept on his front porch: a specially designed double rocker which had two wooden backs with turned dowels, two upholstered seats, two sets of rocking legs, all joined into one unit at the center.

But when the brothers asked their architect to construct a corridor between the two houses with a big room in the center for their study and library, both wives objected. Already the men were together at work all day. When would they have time for their families? The brothers deferred to their wives and settled for a long speaking tube between the houses, so they could signal to one another when they set out for work in the morning.

Naturally, the couples spent a great deal of time together. In 1901 Edith wrote Charlie a letter teasing him about a plan she and Hattie were cooking up for a trip in the future. "Hattie and I think we will go [to California] – won't it be nice? And you and Will can play billiards every night when we are away." Then Edith suggested how Charlie could defeat his brother the next time they played billiards: "Will is planning on doing you up in great shape when you get home. Guess you'll have to take a few lessons of a really scientific player and surprise him – wouldn't it be a joke?"

By the late 1890's the two couples had many friends in and around Rochester and were much in demand for dinners, card parties, and dances. (Edith always loved to dance.) Dr. Charlie and Edith belonged to a formal

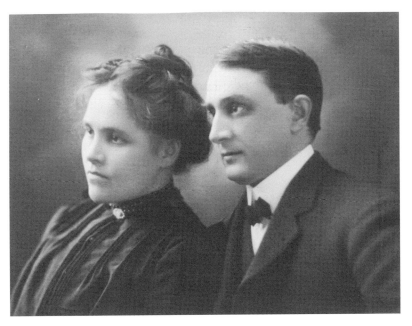

dancing club in those days. A story passed down in the family tells of one night, after an evening out, when Dr. Charlie made a discovery as he undressed. "No wonder I couldn't dance tonight," he said to Edith. "My feet were sticking to the floor. I forgot to take my rubbers off!"

The two Mayo homes, according to Clapesattle, "were among the largest and most comfortably appointed in Rochester" and "jointly [functioned as] a center of the community's social life." In time, because of the doctors' need for family life and for rest, the couples put a stop to the social activity, explaining the dilemma to their many friends. But two or three times a year, one or the other house would hold a dinner or reception for 75, 100, or more – sometimes as many as 300 guests. These parties were important social occasions in Rochester.

Clearly, Edith and Charlie enjoyed people, and because hotel space for visiting doctors in the mid 1890's was limited, the two Mayo homes soon came to be used almost as hotels. Dr. Charlie, especially, liked inviting doctors who had observed his surgeries to his home for lunch or dinner and an overnight stay. Edith had to keep her pantry stocked with plenty of food; she was often asked to serve as many as ten extra dinner guests with almost no advance notice, and to provide them with sleeping accommodations as well. Clapesattle said, "The simple but gracious hospitality ...dispensed has become legendary in medical circles the world over."

In the early days, Edith cooked for the guests herself, using recipes she had learned from her mother. She always enjoyed cooking. Her granddaughter Mayo remembered, "Yes, Granny cooked. Many good things came down from Grahamholm. One was the cookies that were always at Granny's...[with] the wonderful icing on top...molasses cookies .... Also I use her dry dressing each Thanksgiving and Christmas...the very best."

Not only did Edith cook, she also joined eagerly in the

conversation, especially when the guests were doctors. Her confident personality had a positive effect on Charlie, who had been shy as a young man at medical school. His roommate described him in those days as "friendly and pleasant always, though inclined to be somewhat retiring and quiet, with little to say about himself." However, descriptions of him after he married Edith never mention shyness, but rather his humor, warmth and conviviality. Because of these qualities, colleagues at the Clinic learned to seek his assistance with patients who were nervous or difficult in any way. Edith's brother Dr. Kit once asked Dr. Charlie to counsel one of his patients who was so nervous about being pregnant she believed she was going insane. Charlie succeeded, where no one else had, in calming her fears.

Another time, a young woman came to Dr. Charlie convinced she needed brain surgery. He examined her and decided that though there was nothing wrong, she would never accept this diagnosis. Wisely, he admitted her to the hospital, administered some anesthesia, wrapped her head in a bandage, and, when she woke up, told her the problem had been taken care of. She left totally "cured."

Doctors, and especially young doctors taught by Dr. Charlie, have told many humorous stories about him. Once, according to Dr. Chuck, his father examined a hypochondriac; this man complained of every symptom imaginable, except irregular bowels.

Dr. Charlie gave his diagnosis: "I think your problem is constipation."

The patient replied: "But, Doctor Mayo, I have a movement every day."

"Yes," Charlie answered, "I know. But the trouble is — each movement is three days late."

Like Charlie, Edith was known for her own brand of humor, especially clever puns. At parties, she liked to repeat a popular pun of the '90's, toasting her guests with a glass of whatever non-alcoholic beverage was near. (She didn't drink alcohol, because she had often seen her father drink too much.) Lifting her glass, Edith would say, "Champagne to my real friends, and real pain to my sham friends!"

⁓

People who remembered Edith and Charlie's marriage always described their abiding love for one another. Their granddaughter Mayo commented, "One small thing to tell you...the relationship she had with Charlie was about as good as it gets. Mother used to say that she never heard them argue, never a cross word, never a shake of the finger."

Edith's son Dr. Chuck wrote, "My father and Uncle Will both made marriages that were enduring triumphs. It must have contributed significantly to their ability to bear the pressure of their profession. Both marriages were supporting to the brothers, both were filled with affection, respect, and sweetness. I think my mother and father were passionately and romantically in love all their lives. They always slept in a double bed."

⁓

Chapter 4

MOTHERHOOD

The years in the red house began with great sorrow. After enduring the grief of several miscarriages, Edith gave birth to their first full-term baby on March 16, 1895. She was named for Edith's older sister Margaret. The baby lived only five days and died of "inanition," according to her death record. That is, she lacked vigor.

A friend gave Edith a poem by Emma A. Lente to console her on Margaret's death:

A Little One
She was so little when to earth she came,
As helpless as a rose leaf in the wind,
A dainty atom of humanity;
Yet, oh! what love and care she came to find!

She was so little when she went away,
That God's great loving angels must have smiled
On her, and opened swift their sheltering arms
To clasp the tender earth-bud, undefiled.
She was so little. Yet, to hearts that ache
With loss and longing since your hopes were riven,
Rejoice to know those dimpled hands have stretched
A cord unbreakable from earth to heaven.

Months after Margaret died, Edith grew concerned about her much loved mother's health. She wrote Jane Graham on June 23, 1895, from the Palmer House Hotel in Chicago, while accompanying Dr. Charlie on one of his trips to observe surgeries.

"My Dearest Mother —

"...[Charlie's sailboat] is fine. You'll have to have a sail in it this summer.

"Now Mother dear, begin and plan, and I'll assist you, on going up to Waseca with me in two or three weeks — It will just put you on your pins again. Kit's letter said, 'Mother is improving.' I wonder if you have been very ill? I do hope not.

"...Keep well for me, dear Mother. I hate to be away from home when you are not well.

Love to...Kit and Yourself,
Yours, Edith."

That same summer, Edith became an aunt twice over. Her youngest sister, Jennie, gave birth to a son, Donald Graham Williams, and Dinah Graham Olin gave birth to a girl, whom she named Edith, as an expression of love and as consolation to her grieving sister.

Edith's mother did not recover her health; she died on April 16, 1896, three days past her sixty-eighth birthday.

Together, the Mayo brothers and their wives had already endured at least six miscarried babies or infant deaths. Though the men were doctors, they couldn't protect their own families from tragedy.

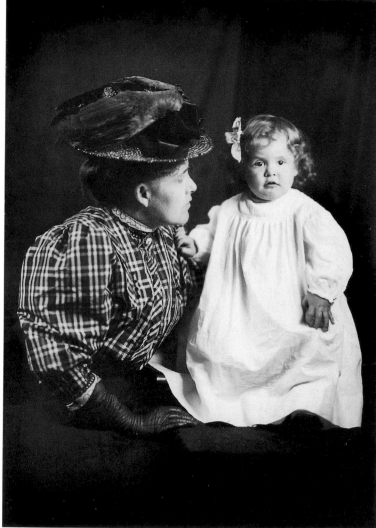

Nobody could.

Then, on January 23, 1897, Edith delivered a second child, healthy and beautiful, and named her Dorothy. Two days later, Hattie gave birth to her daughter Phoebe, named for Will and Charlie's older sister. (This first Phoebe had died at 28, having spent her last seven years a semi-invalid because of an accident. Turning her horse and carriage sharply into the family's driveway one day, she was thrown from the carriage and injured her spleen. At that time, there was no treatment for her. Years later, Dr. Will mastered the surgery which would have saved her life.)

Edith and Hattie delighted together in the robust health of their two precious babies. Living next door to one another, they happily visited often, enjoying the doings and achievements of the little cousins.

On March 11, when Dorothy was nearly seven weeks old, Edith wrote to Dr. Charlie, who was away observing surgeries:

"My dear husband,

"Baby is smiling at me from the cradle — greeting you, perhaps....She grows more beautiful every day, and you will be surprised to find how much she notices....

"I miss you but as long as you are having a good time and Baby is well, I shall not hurry you home.

"Dear, dear husband, I do love you so much and will be glad when you are safely home again. Baby sends a kiss, I, my dearest love,

"Edith."

Though Dorothy brought Edith joy in 1897, two grievous losses that same year brought her sorrow. In late March a letter arrived from her brother Kit with terrible news. Their niece Musetta Graham had been stricken with a fatal illness. He wrote:

"Dear Edith,

"Letters of sadness just received. We have drained the saddest that death can bring, but oh, how deeply this goes to my heart. We love Musie so much, and she [was] always good. How this dread disease got hold mystifies me. I am too broken and sorrowful to write more. How can her nearest own bear it?...

"Sadly,

Kit Graham."

Musetta Graham died on April 8, 1897, at the age of 23. Four months later, Jennie Graham Williams, Edith's youngest sibling, also died, having just turned 25. These losses were unusual in the Graham clan, some of whose members lived into their nineties.

Edith consoled herself with Dorothy, her little nieces Phoebe Mayo and Edith Olin, and her nephew Donald Williams. Before the year was over, she was expecting another child. The two sisters, Edith and Dinah, were pregnant together again in early '98. This time, Dinah gave birth first. Their brother Kit telegraphed Edith in Chicago on March 31, 1898, to give her good news: "Dinah delivered of a girl. O.K." The second Olin daughter was named "Jane," in honor of her recently deceased maternal grandmother.

Four months later, on July 28, 1898, Edith gave birth to her first son, Charles William Mayo, named for his father and his Uncle Will. Dorothy, a bright and affectionate child, was now 18 months old. Edith reveled in being a mother of two.

With Charles's birth, Edith entered a short time of pure, unalloyed happiness. Her two life-long passions were satisfied: she was happy with her family and with the works of healing which she and her husband shared. Being a wife and mother was her delight. Later she told her daughter Louise that "my happiest times were when the children were young and surrounding me. I would often find myself staring at the children, thinking 'They are so beautiful and I love them so much.'"

Edith continued to take pleasure in the growing success of what was called "the Mayos' Clinic." This year her brother Christopher joined the partnership; the practice was growing so fast it soon was in need of another partner, who came the next year, Dr. Melvin C. Millet.

On October 18, 1898, when Baby Charles (later called Chuck) was not yet three months old, Edith wrote Dr. Charlie, speaking of both her interests:

"My darling husband,

"...Dorothy is standing by me trying to kiss the paper, and saying, 'Papa, Papa, I love my papa.' She seems to think this a sort of telephone. We are all as usual well. Had a very good night – Father was down and staid [sic] with me.

"...I may go down to the Congregational Church to supper. Hattie is interested in a tableful but I do feel tired. We have been sweeping the house, and I have been taking care of the babes all day. Had Dorothy and Charles out for a walk, and that is no small job...

"They almost lost a patient with chloroform yesterday. Will says he has used that for the last time....

"The children join me in deep love,

"Yours, Edith."

The only recorded cause for unhappiness this year and the next were the separations Edith and Charlie endured when he traveled to see the newest surgeries. But these trips were a necessity they both accepted. From the beginning of medical practice, Charlie and Will had traveled extensively to learn surgical techniques; usually Charlie did so in the spring and Will in the fall. They were keen to find and practice the very best procedures that would benefit their patients. The Mayo Clinic's motto, "The needs of the patient come first," is an expression of the brothers' great interest in their patients' welfare from the earliest years of their practice.

Dr. Charlie went on a long trip in the early spring of 1899, accompanied by his father. On March 15, he wrote his wife from Chicago. He was concerned about her health:

"My Darling Wife,

"I received yours this noon with Dorothy's enclosed. I thought you [were] feeling bad when I left but imagined that most of it was because I was going away....Put the soap stone on the radiator during the day and then in bed with you at night while your special warmer is away....

"Kiss the little ones for papa, My darling wife,

"Your husband, Chas."

On March 21, Charlie wrote Edith from Baltimore, Maryland, where he and his father had traveled from Chicago. The Doctors Mayo included Baltimore in their itineraries regularly now, in order to observe practices at the new Johns Hopkins Medical School, such as using microscopes to analyze blood and urine in diagnosing diseases, and using rubber gloves during surgery to protect patients from contamination. Although Dr. Charlie found Baltimore a useful center of learning, when he wrote Edith, his thoughts were on his family at home:

"My Darling Wife,

"I have been in to look for my letter a dozen times today, but it may come after supper....How I should like to kiss you, Love, and those dear babies. I bought a doll for Dorothy today, unbreakable, lambs' wool hair. I shall rout out early again to go to Hospital in the morning. Dear wife, I hope your letter will come.

"Kisses to you all,

"Your loving husband, Chas."

The next day, when Dr. Charlie wrote again, he was happy because her letter had arrived. Besides that, he was happy because of the surgeries he had seen: "We had a good day of it – cancer of the breast and lots of skin grafting."

After telling of a prize fight they attended, he mentioned how he missed Edith: "My, how I would like to see you, sweet one. You are the best little mother I know of, but the best wife of all."

In this letter, one can see Dr. Charlie enjoying the luxury of providing well for his family: "I am so glad to hear the children are doing well. Have all the clothes made you need. Don't scrimp yourself, but get what you want. We make more than we can spend anyway now, and we will have the stuff when we bust." (Neither Charlie nor Edith had grown up in households where the rule was "Don't scrimp yourself, but get what you want." Dr. W.W. Mayo didn't bother to collect fees from his patients on a regular basis, so his income was always uncertain until he was joined in his practice by Dr. Will, who collected what was due them. And Edith's father, Joseph Graham, had struggled constantly to support his large family from a small farm.)

Dr. Charlie and his father traveled on to Philadelphia to observe surgeries at German Hospital. On March 24 Charlie wrote Edith,

"I shall...be glad when I start for home. I can see you now, feeding Charles. What a fine mother you are to have such sweet children. But I knew it over 6 years ago. Of course, if it will

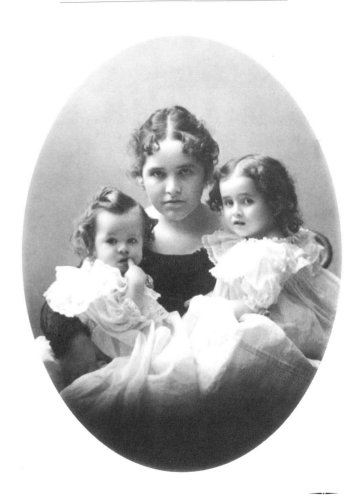

Edith with Dorothy and baby Charles, 1899
Photo courtesy of Olmsted County Historical Society

interrupt the service in the morning, the afternoon will do for a christening. Maybe Charles won't let me hold him when I get back! Kiss the dear little ones, wife, and I will love you always.

"Your loving husband, Chas."

Apparently Dr. Charlie and Edith requested a Sunday morning christening for baby Charles at Calvary Episcopal Church, but changed for the more convenient afternoon time. Both parents were present when Charles was baptized, as they had been for Dorothy. They were communicating members of the church, but whereas Edith went to the 11 a.m. service every Sunday, Dr. Charlie attended irregularly. He worked very long hours and included Sundays in his work week, although with a significant difference: on Sundays he and Dr. Will performed free surgeries for residents of two mental hospitals, one in Rochester and one in St. Peter.

In 1900 Dr. Charlie bought the first automobile in town. It was a light tan four-horsepower steam-powered car with three seats and no top, which could travel as fast as 25 miles an hour. Bertha Wilcox, a young woman from Rochester, saw the thing in operation and said, "Horses were frightened almost beyond control at [its] approach." When Edith was asked years later if she had any photos of that first car, she responded, "No,...but perhaps there are others

about the country [who do], as people were always taking pictures of us when we were stalled, which happened nearly every time Doctor took the car out."

Charlie went on to buy other cars when new models became available. In 1903 he bought an electric auto – also the first in Rochester. Some of these vehicles were shipped to him in boxes, and it was, for him, relaxation to assemble them himself.

Sometime in 1900, Edith's brief period of unmitigated happiness ended. Her dearly loved three-year-old Dorothy contracted scarlet fever and nearly died. The fever shot up so high, Dorothy went into a coma.

Edith had already lost several miscarried babies as well as little Margaret. She was determined not to lose this child. She later told her daughter Louise that she prayed, "Lord, if I never have another child in this world, please let this baby live!"

Then she said to Dorothy, 'You will live! You will live! You will live!' and she placed her in a cold water bath to bring the fever down, then a warm bath, then again the cold water bath.

The fever broke and Dorothy lived, but she was never again mentally normal. According to Mayo Kooiman, "Sometimes [Dorothy] drove all of us crazy....Once she started talking, it was difficult to stop her. But she was capable of many things. The high fever gave her a mentality of – tops – about eight years old. Many things she could not remember, but she was excellent with numbers. Granny always said, 'No need for a telephone book, -- just ask Dorothy.' I used to play canasta with her, game after game after game....

"Granny taught her to always watch what other people did: which spoon to use, which glass to drink from, how to listen to music so she might dance, how to read well enough so she might know where the bathroom was. It was difficult for Granny, who was never left alone."

We have very little record of the suffering Edith endured. Much later, in 1935 when Edith's infant granddaughter, Penelope Trenholm, was desperately ill with pneumonia, Edith alluded to Dorothy's illness. She told the baby's mother, "Louise, I hope, of course, Penny lives. But I will never again pray for a baby to live. There are some things far worse than death. I will never – as much as I hope she lives – pray for a baby to live." (Penny did live.)

For Dr. Charlie, there was a practical solution to his grief some years later. Just as Dr. Will became an expert in spleen surgery after his sister Phoebe died of a spleen injury, so Charlie devoted himself to ridding Rochester of scarlet fever in 1912, years after Dorothy's illness. There was then no full-time public health officer in Rochester. When scarlet fever struck in epidemic numbers, and even two visiting surgeons contracted it, Dr. Charlie rounded up women from the Civic League one night and with their help presented a strong case before the city council,

asking that a capable officer be hired. The city council discussed the matter such a long time that Dr. Charlie went home to bed. About one-thirty a.m., loud knocks on his door awoke him. It was the city council, ready to swear him in as health officer, even in his pajamas and robe. Immediately, Dr. Charlie quarantined all scarlet fever cases in their homes and ended the epidemic.

⌒

Life continued in the red house. Another baby was born to Edith and Dr. Charlie on October 20, 1900, and named for her – Edith. She was a sweet baby. Growing up, she more and more resembled her mother – very pretty, with dark brown eyes and dark brown hair.

On November 4, Edith wrote to Dr. Charlie at the Briggs House, a hotel in Chicago where he was staying on one of his surgery inspection trips. She had heard from him that he was having a good time with the doctors, and this made her happy: "It is a good opportunity to get well acquainted with the famous men of medicine and surgery – and I am so glad you are there to meet and be met."

Baby Edith was only fifteen days old. Both she and her mother were doing well: "I have been up much of the day and took a bath in the tub alone this A.M....so you see I am getting strong very rapidly – and Baby is just as good as pie, and nurses only once in the night." But this letter also tells of the separation sadness Dorothy was experiencing. "Dorothy began to sniffle last night and say,

'I want my papa – I want my papa to come back.'"

By March 26, 1901, Dorothy was four years old, little Charles two and a half, and the baby five months. Edith wrote to her husband, away in Chicago again, "The children are too gay for anything. Sophia [a household helper] is just starting over to Phoebe's with Charles in a blanket, and Dorothy is watching out of window [sic] for her return, when she is going over. Yesterday we promised they might go over, and instead Hattie and Phoebe came here, and Dorothy set up such a roar and wanted her to go home so she and Charles might visit over there."

Dorothy remained over-excitable her whole life. This letter is the first mention of a person hired to help with the children – Sophia. In the next letter, written two days later, Edith mentioned Mary, who had given notice that she could work for them only a few more weeks. Because of this, Edith was advertising in the weekly paper for another helper.

After Dorothy's illness, Edith didn't sleep well when Charlie was away. She ends the letter, *"I had a horribly lonely wakeful night. I don't know what possessed me, but sleep I could not....*

"My love, Your love,
"Edith."

Two days later, on March 28, Edith wrote her husband in St. Louis, Missouri, about the new baby and also about her sleep problem:

"My darling husband,

"The old babies have been asleep hours, but the new baby has just left my arms. I am afraid she is not going to be such a good youngster anymore. She is beginning to know altogether too much, and shows an inclination to run things which I do not wish to pamper, but I am frequently forced to concede a good bit to her wishes.... I miss you so, and somehow cannot rest at all in the night. I begin to feel lonely at twilight and am so glad for the mornings. It makes me tired but I can't help it."

Edith decided to solve an old problem in a new way. Whenever Charlie traveled, the separation caused grief to husband and wife, as well as to the children. Now, Edith made plans to leave the children with their caregivers and join Charlie in Chicago. Leaving the children was hard for Edith. Jane Twentyman Graham had always been a hands-on, stay-at-home mother, and Edith's instincts were to emulate her. But Edith was practical; she accepted as inevitable her need for household help, because without it she could not handle the scope of entertaining which Charlie wanted her to do. She knew the continual dinner parties and overnight guests benefited Charlie, helping him learn from, and teach, other doctors. Also, Edith felt she could help Charlie by traveling with him occasionally. So she wrote him:

"Today I had Carl bring down our mammoth trunk, and when I look at it and think of the old babies, I

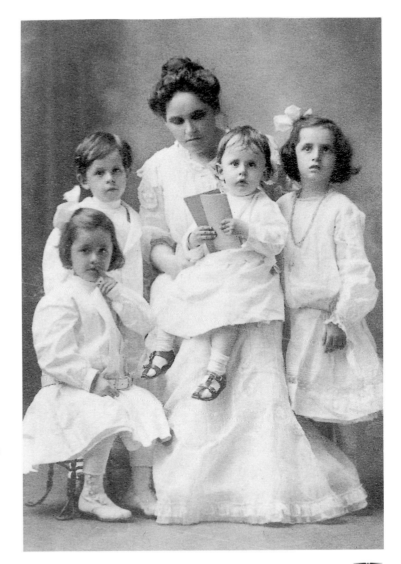

tremble, and when I think of you, my heart sings. I shall be so glad to meet you. I am no good alone."

She mentioned the other subject dear to her heart – work at the Clinic: "I had a nice letter from Dr. Prince yesterday. He said he had never seen better surgery than in Rochester and doubted if it existed."

Then she concluded, "Well, my darling boy, I must say goodnight – and hie me to my lonely couch."

As time went by, Edith traveled with Dr. Charlie more and more, whenever she thought the children could bear her absence.

Another son was born, Joseph Graham Mayo, on August 31, 1902. The new baby was named for his maternal grandfather, a widower who lived on for another twelve years. Little Joe is always described as humorous and fun-loving.

By this time the household staff in the red house was growing. (The Mayos, with an eye for the dignity of persons, never referred to those who worked for them as "servants." They were "staff.") In the 1905 census, persons living in the red house – besides Dr. Charlie, Edith and the four children – were a 38-year-old governess from Germany, another woman from Germany (Anna Newman, who was 22 at this time), and two other women, listed as "domestics." Anna remained with the family 38 more years, helping with the children and, when they were grown, acting as head housekeeper.

On August 21, 1905, Edith gave birth to another daughter, Louise, who was named for her paternal grandmother. Louise's beautiful, naturally-curly brown hair was always a special delight to her mother, whose own darker brown hair was straight. Like her older sister Edith, Louise had big, dark brown eyes.

During these years when Dr. Charlie's family was growing, the "Mayos' Clinic" was growing too. In 1901 William Beck Graham, Edith's oldest brother, was hired as office manager, leaving his previous work as overseer of cheese factories in Rochester and St. Paul. Dr. E. Starr Judd joined the Mayo practice in 1902, after graduating from the University of Minnesota Medical School. Edith and Dr. Charlie had befriended him by then; in fact, Edith took him into the red house during the summers while he was at medical school . Judd's mother had died, leaving him no home in Rochester, and Edith, realizing this, invited him to live with them. According to Dr. Judd's daughter, Eleanor Judd Kirklin, "Aunt Edith always had her hands out to help somebody."

By 1906, Dr. Stinchfield had retired from the practice, but (besides Dr. Will, Dr. Charlie, Dr. Kit Graham and Dr. Millet,) Dr. Henry S. Plummer had joined as a partner. Dr. Will said that "hiring…Henry Plummer was the best day's work [I] ever did for the Clinic," and he called Plummer "the best brain the Clinic ever had."

Some of the doctors who joined the Mayo practice at this time came as research assistants, for ever since their childhoods, when their father mortgaged his farm to buy a microscope, Will and Charlie had understood the importance of research to the successful treatment of patients. On January 1, 1905, the gifted pathologist Dr. Louis B. Wilson began work for the Drs. Mayo. One day soon after, Dr. Will told him, "I wish you…would find a way to tell us surgeons whether a growth is cancer or not while the patient is still on the table." At that time, tissues taken from patients were routinely hardened in alcohol before being placed under the microscope, a process which took some time. On an extremely cold January morning, Wilson came up with a new idea. He placed fresh tissue samples outside on a windowsill; they froze quickly and he stained them with methylene blue dye so they could be analyzed in minutes. This was a breakthrough discovery which enabled surgeons to diagnose and repair in just one operation. Today, the Mayo Clinic tissue collection is one of the world's largest and is vital to medical research.

The Mayo brothers continued to take annual trips to other surgical arenas. By the beginning of the twentieth century, though, outstanding doctors had also begun visiting them. In 1901 Great Britain's foremost surgeon, Dr. Arthur Robson, spent a week observing Dr. Will and Dr. Charlie at the Clinic; and in 1903, the leading surgeon of all Europe, Dr. Johann von Mikulicz-Radecki, came from Breslau, Germany, to watch the brothers at work. In 1905, Dr. Dudley Tait of San Francisco told the American Surgical Association, "I have journeyed to Rochester, to that great surgical shrine where dominate two masters, and on each occasion of my pilgrimage...I have come away bewildered with a knowledge of what I saw there. I have carried that knowledge to my masters in Europe, and they shared my enthusiasm for the work done at Rochester."

Since the 1890's, Dr. Will had been delivering medical papers at surgical conventions, representing both brothers. The brothers decided in the early 1900's that Dr. Charlie must become a speaker too. He was reluctant at first, believing that because he spoke slowly and organized his thoughts more intuitively and less logically than his brother, he could not present their work as well. So Edith helped him. They began working together on his speeches. He would write a speech and then practice it with her, sometimes many times – until midnight or after.

On speech night, Edith would go along, planning to indicate by hand signals if Charlie needed to speak louder, softer, faster, slower. If Edith raised her handkerchief above her eye level, it meant, "Speak up!" According to Clapesattle, who heard the story directly from Edith, "Poor Mrs. Mayo was always disconcerted. She never heard the speech they had so carefully prepared and rehearsed, because Dr. Charlie simply could not stick to his manuscript. He would think of something extra to say or some story he wanted to tell and would soon be so far from the prepared speech that there was no use trying to get back to it." Clapesattle added, "Dr. Charlie's charm as a speaker is still a byword with all who knew him. His chuckle-raising humor and his droll stories are legendary in Rochester and in medical circles the country over."

On June 3, 1906, Dr. Charlie and his brother-in-law Dr. Graham traveled to Boston to a meeting of the American Surgical Society where Dr. Charlie was a speaker. Kit wrote his sister a glowing account of the evening:

"My dear Edith:

"I have been intending to write you since...Charlie so signally made his impress on the American Surgical Society. Without flattery for him or you, just pure admiration for him, and the knowledge that a loving wife is always glad to hear of

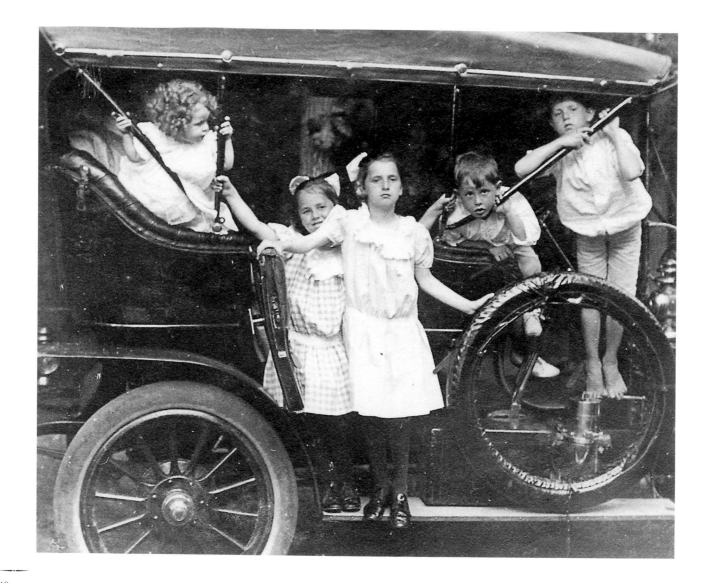

the honest achievements of a husband, do I write you much of this. In Cleveland, among staff of the surgical profession of this and other countries, Charlie shone undoubtedly as one of first magnitude – clear and rapid in delivery, every word and every sentence heard and appreciated, his paper was the best and received as such. His discussion the following day was terse, pointed, scientific, and bountifully and beautifully commented upon, – his big round black eyes just shone, and he seemed lifted from himself and living in quite a different sphere....He had the fire and force necessary and carried the meeting with as much certainty as I had seen Will at other times, but in his own peculiar way was Charlie distinctive....But Charlie needs neither me nor other person to speak, he can and has done for himself and Oh! I was proud....Grab him and hug him and tell him of your just pride in your small but large and great blackeyed surgeon....Will and Charlie are a pair and both are equally famous, each in his own peculiar, personal way. It is good to see earned greatness, properly appreciated, and Will and Charlie are surely in the surgical zenith today."
This letter Edith kept and treasured her entire life.

Dr. Charlie continued to progress as a surgeon. Whereas Dr. Will was by now specializing in surgery of the abdomen (appendix, gall bladder, stomach, spleen), Dr. Charlie had always maintained diverse specialties. He operated on the eye, thyroid, spinal column, prostate, – whatever was not inside the abdomen. The diversity of his skills and the ingeniousness of his surgical solutions to problems prompted their colleague Dr. Haggard to say: "Dr. Will is a wonderful surgeon, but Dr. Charlie is a surgical wonder."

Dr. Charlie's daughter Louise also described him in colorful terms. As a little girl, she didn't understand what her father did for a living. But she remembered hearing her mother say he worked like a dog. If someone asked what her father was doing, she'd say, "working like a dog."

On January 10, 1908, thirteen days before Dorothy's eleventh birthday, Edith gave birth to another daughter, whom they named Rachel. She had brown hair and beautiful clear blue eyes, the only one of Edith's children with blue eyes.

Dr. Charlie's children all adored him. At lunchtime, he used to come home to the red house to eat with his family. One day a visitor, noticing how the littlest children were climbing all over their father, remarked to Edith that it was too bad Charlie wasn't able to nap at this time, since he had performed so many surgeries in the morning and still

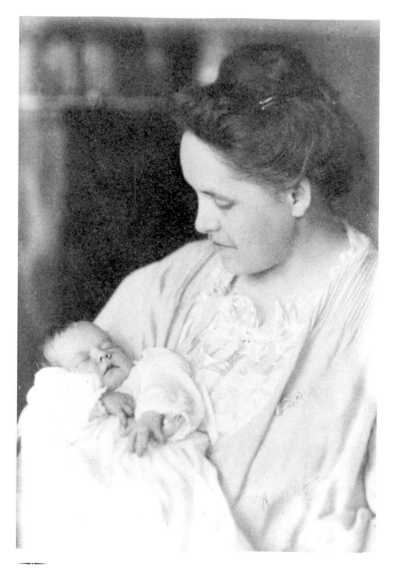

had more to go.

"Look at him more closely," Edith suggested. Then the visitor noticed that Dr. Charlie was asleep—-he had trained himself to nap in the midst of his children's activity.

During these years in the red house, Edith continued entertaining out-of-town doctors and patients, as she had been doing since the mid-1890's. This became a settled feature of her life with Charlie. Her daughter Louise said, "Practically never were we alone at dinner."

But on Sundays, the family enjoyed a ride into the country when the weather was fine. Dr. Charlie would take Edith and the children in an open car, with a team of horses and a wagon following behind, in case the car broke down. Their destination was about twelve miles away, near Oronoco, a house converted into a restaurant where delicious home cooking was served. Chicken with dumplings and lots of gravy was the specialty. After enjoying a big dinner together, the family would continue their Sunday drive.

Another place for fun was the summer house on the lake near Oronoco which Dr. Charlie owned jointly with his brother. In the summertime, the brothers rotated weeks of residency. Here the main amusements were

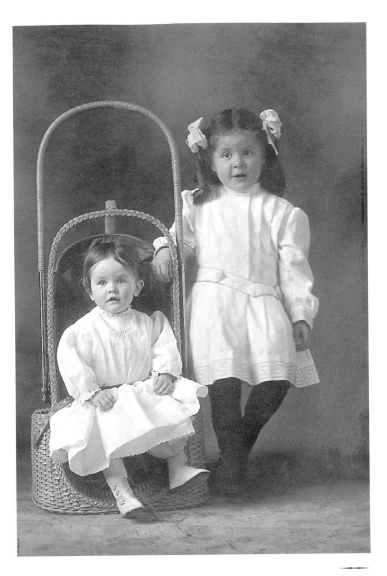

swimming and boating. Dr. Charlie, always fascinated
with mechanical things, liked to put motor launches
together. Once, he rigged up a launch and invited
Edith, with her picnic hamper, aboard for the first
excursion. Dr. Charlie pushed the boat free from shore
and turned on the motor. He soon discovered, when
the boat made for shore, that he had installed the motor
backwards. Calmly, Dr. Charlie turned the boat
around, and he and Edith enjoyed their trip across the
lake just as planned, only stern first.

Daughter Edith remembered Dr. Charlie's
excitement about animals and how he would waken the
children if something interesting happened at night. At
Oronoco late one night, he woke all the children,
according to Edith, "and told us to hurry up outside -
that he'd found flying squirrels. We all rushed out in our
nighties."

As the Clinic grew, accounting and bookkeeping
became a job for more than one man. Therefore, in
1908 Harry Harwick joined Edith's brother William
Beck Graham in the business office. Like Dr. Plummer,
Harwick was an innovator; he gradually introduced an
up-to-date record-keeping system.

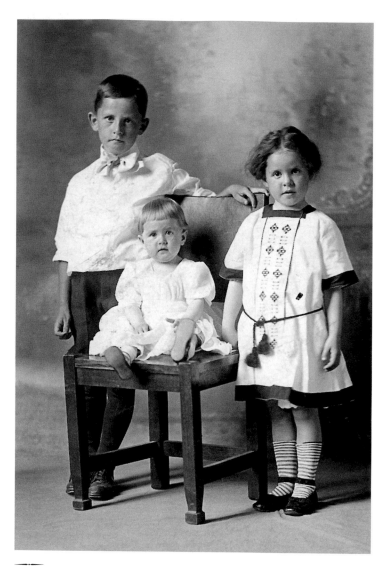

Joe with baby Esther and Louise in 1909

Photo courtesy of Mayo Kooiman

Edith delivered another daughter, Esther, the last of her eight children, on April 2, 1909. This little one had hazel eyes and straight hair like her mother, though of a lighter brown. A fun-loving little girl, she was later described by her elder brother Chuck as an "imp," full of mischief.

A great sorrow occurred in the family the following year, just past Esther's first birthday. Rachel, two years old, died on May 28, 1910. Her death was neither sudden nor unexpected, since she had been in poor health for some months. Though Edith and Dr. Charlie did all they could, the child died anyway of "ileocolitis," according to her death certificate, which Dr. Charlie signed. This condition is an inflammation of the lowest division of the small intestine.

In early June Edith received a letter from a friend, Mrs. Oviatt: "It is with my deepest sympathy that I write you this letter, for I know how full of sorrow your own dear heart is. Only such devoted mothers as yourself can feel the loss of such a delicate flower child as was the dear little Rachel. I was not surprised, my dear, for I felt sure when I saw her in February, that she could not be with you long, and my heart ached then for the little blossom."

Rachel's bronzed baby shoes and her silver baby spoon were kept as treasures in the family. Edith also kept a toy which Rachel had especially liked, a little white woolen lamb with blue eyes and a blue ribbon with a tiny golden bell tied around its neck. Later, even after Edith moved from the red house, this lamb still stood on a shelf in her room. More than 20 years after Rachel's death, Edith's little granddaughter Muff asked to play with the lamb.

"Granny would let me hold it for awhile," Muff wrote, "but although I would beg her to let me have it, she wouldn't. She always said, 'That was Rachel's.'

"'Who is Rachel and where is she?' I would ask."

"Granny would always answer me quietly, 'Rachel died, but she loved this very much, so hold it now, but then we will put it back.'"

It may have been at the time of Rachel's death that Edith came to rely on what later became one of her favorite and most repeated sayings, "Thy will be done!" Both her granddaughter Muff and her grandson Charles Rankin remembered her saying this or a variation, "It's God's will!" She came to understand that by accepting an accomplished grief, and seeing it as part of a larger divine plan, she could move on and live eagerly and confidently in the present moment again.

Little Rachel died on the same day a happy event occurred in the extended family – Dr. Will and Hattie's older daughter Carrie married Dr. Donald C. Balfour in a beautiful wedding performed in the yellow house, next door to Edith and Dr. Charlie. Dr. Balfour was already a surgeon on the Clinic staff. Four years after his wedding, he was made a partner in the Mayo practice, the last partner.

Edith and Dr. Charlie mastered their grief and attended the wedding, being careful not to tell anyone of Rachel's death. When Carrie and Dr. Balfour discovered this, while on their honeymoon in Toronto, Canada, they both wrote letters expressing their thanks and love. Dr. Balfour wrote,
"My Dear Aunt,

"...That such a grief should enter your home in the same hour that Carrie and I were so proudly showing our happiness to the world, seems cruel. Then, in the face of your sorrow, to have such consideration for us that the sadness at your home was kept from us, and at such a time that you and Dr. Charlie should come over and give us your blessings---well, we shall never forget it.

"Lovingly yours,
"Donald."

That same year, 1910, an important event happened: the family began construction of a large house on the country property they called "Mayowood." Dr. Charlie had purchased a hilly, wild, wooded platte bordering the Zumbro River in 1900. At first the family used it

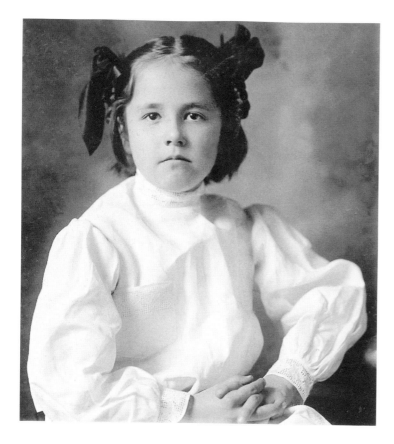

Daughter Edith at age 10 in 1910

Photo courtesy of Edith Rankin Redden

mostly for picnics, which were memorable family outings because of Dr. Charlie's amazing knowledge of plants and animals. He loved telling the children stories about nature.

On one of these picnics, to celebrate Chuck's eighth birthday in 1906, the family gathered around a big oak tree on a lovely level piece of land which backed into a large hill. Dr. Charlie began describing the big house he would like to build there. He walked around the site, putting sticks in the ground and unwinding twine in room-size squares and rectangles to show how he would design the house.

Between 1900 and 1910, Dr. Charlie conducted farming experiments on his country property, and, as adjoining farms became available for sale, he bought them. Eventually, he owned more than 3,000 acres. He also hired workers to build a cottage for weekend retreats which he and Edith named "the Ivy Cottage." Its mode of construction was his own idea: poured concrete walls with an insulating air space between, designed so the house would retain coolness in summer, and heat in winter. Dr. Charlie was so pleased with the project he decided to undertake a more lavish enterprise — construction of a big house which followed exactly the design he had set for it four years earlier.

Chapter 5

REARING A FAMILY AT MAYOWOOD

By 1910, Dr. Charlie had mastered the intricacies of thyroid surgery, but he could not explain to other surgeons why he operated one way on one patient, another way on another. Neither could Dr. Plummer, who worked closely with him. The pathology had not yet caught up to what Dr. Charlie understood intuitively. Consequently, many doctors came to observe him in thyroid surgery, but instead of copying his techniques, they referred their cases to him. The streets of Rochester were beginning to fill with so many strange-looking goiter patients that, according to Clapesattle, "pregnant women in Rochester were afraid to go downtown lest they mark their babies by their repugnance at the sight of the many big necks and protruding eyeballs."

Thyroid operations increased from 1000 per year to 5000 per year in four years; they became the most frequent operation at the Mayo Clinic. Dr. Charlie was earning well from all this labor. Yet neither he nor Dr. Will had ever been motivated toward surgery by a love for money. In fact, they generously gave free surgeries to the poor. After the First World War, theirs was the first clinic in America to routinely give free medical care to veterans, an effort which in time led to the creation of veterans' hospitals.

At one point, the Drs. Mayo even considered cutting their surgical fees, because of too much money left in their common purse at year's end. But they felt it would be unfair to neighboring doctors if they undercut them. So in 1900 Dr. Will and Dr. Charlie began to invest their left-over funds, using the counsel of a wise Rochester attorney, Burt W. Eaton. By 1910 there was enough money in the account for Dr. Charlie to indulge in a beautiful, original house for his large family. He built it of poured concrete with insulating air spaces, like Ivy Cottage.

"The house caused quite a stir in Rochester," Dr. Chuck later reported. It has been said to be in the tradition of Frank Lloyd Wright, the "Prairie School style," because the structure looks like a rocky outcropping with walls more than one foot thick, growing out of a large hill. But it is really in no particular style at all except Dr. Charlie style.

In the original house were eight bathrooms and more than thirty rooms altogether, including a living room of 1,200 square feet and a ballroom even larger. Eventually, a small elevator was installed, which could take people from ground level to the fourth or ballroom floor or one floor higher, atop the house, where an observatory held a big swing. This was a favorite place for family and friends to admire the spacious view of the Zumbro River Valley below.

Garfield Schwartz, the contractor, hired 30 men to construct the house; he also bought the largest concrete mixer ever used in Rochester to make the wall material. Dr. Chuck said, "Father reinforced the concrete with old scythes and plowshares from the local junkyard; we could

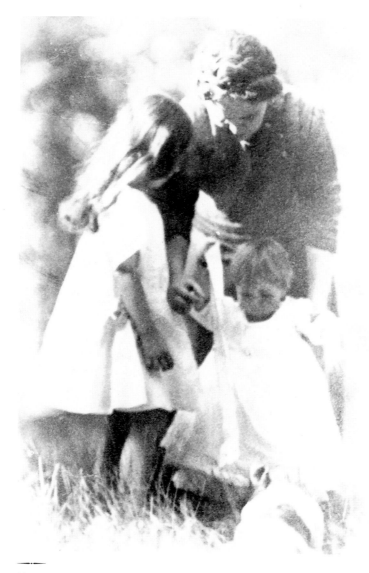

Edith helping Esther to walk,
with Louise standing by to assist in 1910

Photo courtesy of Mayo Kooiman

withstand a siege in Mayowood."

The first cool air system in the area was built for the house. On hot days, a pump pulled chilly air from cabins in the back hillside into the house. Also a powerful vacuum made life easier for the household staff. Each room had a hole which could be fitted with a hose. When the machine was turned on, dirt was sucked into a room in the basement.

Though the house was imposing, Edith made sure it kept the country look she loved. "Everywhere there were touches of simplicity," Mayo said. There were "pots full of geraniums, a few hollyhocks, and...sweetpeas climbing and hanging on the stone walls."

Later the family added a tea house, a front terrace on the ground floor, and a curving entrance drive which was bordered by an English-style "dragon tooth" stone wall. Dr. Charlie caused the Zumbro River to be excavated and dammed, creating a beautiful lake in the valley which could be seen from the long living room and front terrace. Then he built arched Oriental bridges, connecting islands in the lake to the shore, and a bath house with solar heated water on the largest island. Together, Dr. Charlie and Edith bought fountains and stone lanterns, so that, according to Dr. Chuck, "on a summer night, it was breath-taking. It helped that he was building in the days before the tax on income."

To provide electricity, Dr. Charlie built a small hydroelectric plant on the Zumbro River. This project required much inventiveness and patience: it took 12 attempts to erect a successful dam. For times of low water or a frozen river, Dr. Charlie bought a very large gasoline generator. In addition to all these improvements, he built a big greenhouse, and a racetrack and stables for their horses.

Wild animals lived on the property too. A pen held small royal Japanese deer, which were, in Muff's words, "the gift of some G.P. – Grateful Patient." When another G.P., an Indian chief, gave Dr. Charlie a white buffalo, another pen was built down by the river. The buffalo eventually had company – a pair of white deer of an African species, gift of another patient. Other animals lived in a third pen – one was Topsey, a black bear cub which Dr. Charlie brought back from a fishing trip; Topsey grew up and was sent to the Bronx Zoo. Besides these penned animals, wild elk and Minnesota whitetail deer roamed the area, so Dr. Charlie built a large fence to keep them out.

Moving into the new home, which the family called "the Big House," was an adventure for them all. For Edith, the new location meant great change. Daily life was far more complex than in town. Even a simple task like calling the children for dinner was more

difficult: with so much space for their roaming, they couldn't hear the sound of a voice. Edith installed a giant dinner bell on a wall behind the house and created a system of signals for meals. The first strike of the bell was a warning – "Come in!" The second strike, some minutes later, meant, "Dinner is almost ready," and the third strike – if you heard it while still outside, too bad for you.

In the red house, Edith had been within walking distance of the Clinic, Calvary Church, and many friends and family, including her father. In the country, no one was handy. To reach town required a car and chauffeur on fine days; on muddy or snowy days, better stay home. This meant Edith created amusements for the children when they couldn't be with town friends. Often, she brought these friends to Mayowood for weekend visits instead.

She didn't mind the complication of her life, because she and the children loved the outdoors and the opportunities to ride horses. Best of all, Dr. Charlie found country life just what he needed to relax from the stress of surgery. He loved to roam over his property, preferably accompanied by at least one child, and check what was happening. Which fences needed mending and why? How many wild geese stopped at the feeding spot? Were the little Japanese deer doing well?

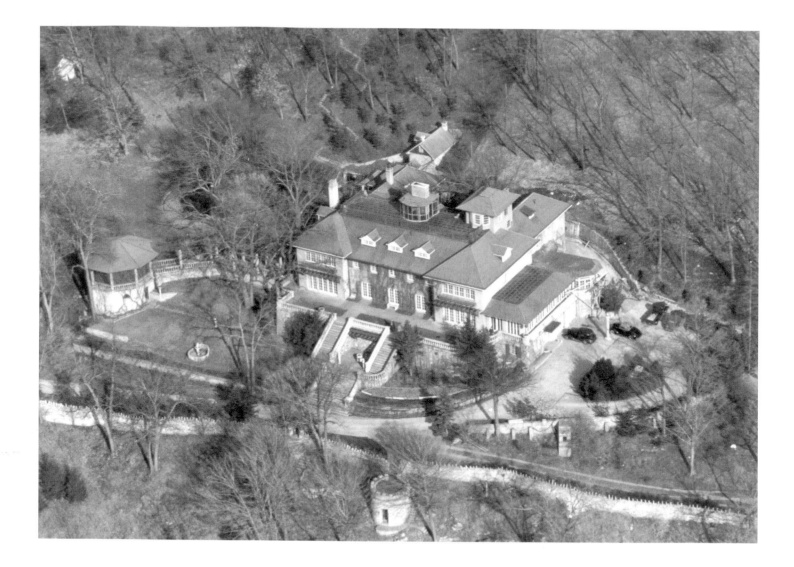

The Clinic was growing at a great rate during these years. Between 1908 and 1912 the number of patients tripled. It grew so rapidly it became an entity in Edith's life – almost like a living creature, whose needs she began to give high priority. Later, when Dr. Chuck married, Edith expressed the importance she had for years been assigning the Clinic. Edith told Dr. Chuck's fiancee, "You're going to do just as I did, exactly. You'll find you haven't married a Mayo, you've married the Mayo Clinic. Remember, the Clinic will always come first [in your husband's life], then you, then your children."

She was stating the priorities she believed Alice should assume when she married, because 34 years of marriage to Dr. Charlie had taught her these were the right priorities. To Edith and Dr. Charlie, the Clinic ranked first because healing the sick was a God-inspired service. Edith considered medicine the greatest calling in the world, even greater than the pastor's calling. "A doctor's calling is a sacred calling," she had said. Under the Clinic in rank Edith put her passionate attachment to her family – her husband first, and then her children. At least that was her official position. Only twice was she unable to live out this creed of putting the Clinic

first – when it meant loss to her beloved brother Dr. Kit and again much later to her beloved son-in-law Dr. Fred Rankin.

As hostess of Mayowood, Edith operated the Big House – as she had the red house – as both a warm haven full of fun for her family and also a quasi-hotel for doctors and out-of-town friends visiting the Clinic. A patient-friend from Philadelphia, Pennsylvania, wrote Edith a note of thanks that testifies to the Mayos' pleasant hospitality: "It was a joy to me – every moment I was at Mayowood – it always is, and because of it, I never mind anything at the Clinic. The worst thing that could happen to me – I'd try to bear pleasantly – -because I'd hate so to go back on you two wonderful people. So that's how I feel. It was heavenly and seems now like a beautiful dream."

A doctor from Australia described a dinner at Mayowood which he and two other doctors enjoyed: "Charles Mayo…called for me in his car.…It was a lovely frosty moonlight night. We drove up to a fine 'cement' house…on the side of a hill overlooking a valley, in which there is a winding river looking very beautiful in the moonlight.…His wife is a charming lady. We had an old-fashioned tea-dinner…all very plain and homely; …His wife joked him about the farm, especially about a flock of geese, of which he was proud, but which had—-so she said—-that day flown away. So he told us about his farm experiences.…His is a charmingly simple home and household – he a delightful personality."

Edith enjoyed leading the dinner talk to amusing subjects, especially gentle teasing of her husband. Surgeons were frequent dinner guests; Dr. Charlie was a friend and host, over the years, to hundreds of doctors. He and Dr. Will were original members of a club of forty outstanding surgeons who met at one or another surgical center to learn from each other, the Society of Clinical Surgery. Besides this, there was the Rochester Surgeons Club for the benefit of doctors who came to observe at the Mayo Clinic. By the end of August, 1906, the same year it was organized, more than 300 doctors had joined the club, and, according to Clapesattle, "the roster…reads like a medical roll call of the American states, the Canadian provinces, and many foreign lands."

On February 2, 1911, Dr. William Worrall Mayo and Louise Wright Mayo observed their sixtieth wedding anniversary, which they celebrated with a family party. At that time they were the longest-married couple in Olmsted County. Dr. Mayo's poor health diminished the merriment of everyone present. More than a year earlier he had absent-mindedly stuck his left arm in a shucking machine at his farm to free a stuck corncob.

Edith on a chaise lounge, reading to her children and Dr. Charlie in 1912

from left, standing: Daughter Edith, Joe, Dr. Charlie, Chuck

from left, seated: Dorothy, Louise, Esther, Edith

Photo courtesy of Olmsted County Historical Society

His fingers were badly crushed. According to Dr. Chuck, Dr. Will examined the injured hand at the Clinic and "said something to the effect that anyone who knew as much about farming as Grandfather did should have better sense than to put his hand in a corn shucker. With that, Grandfather exploded and ordered him out of the room. 'Only Charlie will take care of me!' he shouted." So Dr. Charlie operated on him.

Three more operations were performed in 1910, the last one to amputate the hand and forearm. The injury caused the old doctor constant pain. Six weeks past his anniversary, he died, leaving another void in Edith's life, for she had maintained a steadfast friendship with him from the day he hired her, never minding that she was "too young and too beautiful" to be a nurse.

In the late autumn of 1911, Dr. Charlie and Edith traveled to Washington, D.C., so he could attend a Southern Surgical Association meeting. From there they traveled on to New York City, where Dr. Charlie suddenly became sick. He self-diagnosed his problem

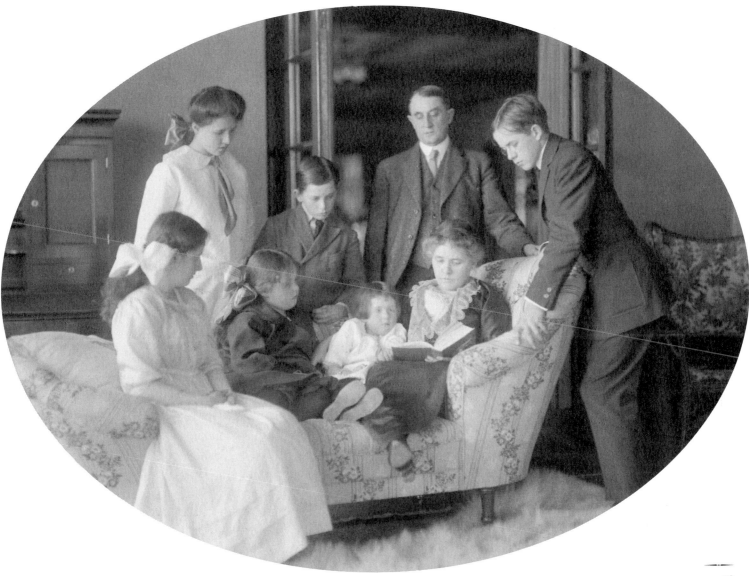

as gallstones, but the N.Y.C. surgeon who attended him disagreed and removed Dr. Charlie's appendix.

After this, Dr. Charlie remained gravely ill – in danger of dying. Dr. Will received news of his brother's condition at 4 a.m. on a cold December morning. In half an hour, he and Dr. Charlie's nurse-anesthetist, Florence Henderson, were on a locomotive, speeding to Winona, where a train was prepared – a "special," which was given precedence over other trains on a record-breaking trip to New York. Newspapers across the country carried the story of the famous Dr. Will rushing to the bedside of his desperately ill brother, the famous Dr. Charlie.

Following an operation to remove his gallbladder, the real source of the problem, Dr. Charlie recovered. Slowly he gained strength, and in January, 1912, he and Edith were able to return to Rochester, where they celebrated a late Christmas with their greatly relieved and overjoyed children.

Edith was living according to her priorities, putting the Mayo Clinic first, her husband second, her children third. Travel with Charlie became a regular part of her life after they moved to Mayowood. She could do this with an easy conscience, trusting her household helpers to watch over the children, and also her larger Graham family to rally round them while she was away. Edith's sister Margaret Twentyman, who frequently moved into the Big House to be with the children when Edith was

traveling, wrote to her and Charlie in 1912:
"Dear ones,

"Just a line to say everybody well. Miss Wilson and I were out to the farm today and had such a good time. The children were so pleased to see us. We played with all till after dinner, then when the little girls [Louise and Esther] were taking their nap, Joseph took us through the woods to the log house. He is a dandy boy, good as gold.... Wish I could have staid [sic] but Esther wanted [me] too. She clung to me all the time. I got lots of kisses and hugs, so you see it made me happy. Joseph always has hugs and kisses for me when you are away. Esther did not want me to wear your hat. She said 'that is my dear mama's.'"

Little Esther's insecurities were no doubt assuaged the following year, as life at Mayowood assumed its normal course. In the summer of 1913, Dorothy was sixteen; Chuck about to turn fifteen; Edith twelve; Joe ten, going on eleven; Louise seven, going on eight, and Esther four. Edith made sure something interesting was always happening for the children. She promoted learning. Teachers came to the house for dancing and piano lessons. Some of the children benefitted more than others: Young Edith, Louise, and Esther enjoyed playing the piano, but Chuck had little aptitude for it. Although he practiced dutifully, his only memorized piece was "The Happy Farmer," which he played, by his own report "doggedly in recital after recital, with decreasing effect."

Edith enjoyed music and at one time wanted a grand piano at Mayowood.

"We have so many guests, Charlie," she pointed out. "It would make entertaining so nice."

Her grandson Charles Rankin described what happened: "Granddad would not hear of it. Too expensive. Too big. Unnecessary. Over and over Granny's plea was turned down.

"One day Granddad came home and delightedly said, 'Edith! Guess what! I just bought a boat for the family to use traveling up and down the Mississippi River. Isn't that great? And, Edith, I'm going to let you name it. What shall we call it?'

"'Baby Grand,' said Granny.

"That indeed became the name of the boat, and the next day a baby grand piano was delivered to Mayowood!"

Not only did the family play on Baby Grand piano, but the famous Finnish composer, Jan Sibelius, played on it too. Esther, when she was very young, sat on his lap and remembered he had a bald head and solid gold teeth. He also brought along a little man to turn the pages of his music.

Another source of music which became increasingly popular with the family as time went by was an aeolian organ which was installed in a room next to the living room in 1913, turning this little entrance chamber into "the music room."

In addition to dancing and music, Dr. Charlie encouraged the children to develop mechanical abilities, which were abundant in him. He designed surgery tools, the first surgery table and a hydraulic elevator at St. Mary's, and innumerable improvements for farming and household life. One of daughter Edith's fondest memories, when she was in her early teens, was of playing with a radio under Dr. Charlie's eye in a room where he kept a shelf full of radio parts. (He had one of the first radios in Rochester.) She said, "I could go up there and twist knobs, and I'd get so excited about being able to hear things!" Later, as an adult, Edith loved working with her hands, and she brought gadgets of all kinds into her home.

Edith and Dr. Charlie encouraged their children in art as well. When Louise was six, soon after the family moved to Mayowood, her father gave her a large chunk of modeling clay. She was thrilled. She worked with it hour after hour. Soon Louise was turning out interesting objects from her fascinating clay. Dr. Charlie liked her work so well that when company came, he would ask her to bring out art projects for the guests to admire. (This early fun with clay was so important to Louise, she grew up to be a sculptor.)

Louise also liked cats and at one time had 23 of them. They slept in holes in the hill behind the house. But so many cats meant trouble for the purple martins that swooped about eating mosquitoes in the late summer afternoons. So Dr. Charlie offered Louise the first real money she had ever earned: one dollar per cat, the cats being distributed to other places around the countryside. Reluctantly, Louise handed over 21 animals, keeping only a mother cat and an old cat which had fits. These two were given collars and bells; the birds had fair warning if they were being hunted.

Edith's children always loved the outdoors, especially riding horses. On weekends, a groom would bring the family's horses from the stables early; some holidays everyone would rise at six for a brisk before-breakfast ride. The whole family, except maybe the youngest baby, would ride together along gravel paths through the woods. Louise remembered riding with the others when she was so small she was mounted on a Shetland pony.

Edith never lost her childhood love of horses. She wrote her son Chuck in 1914, when she was 47, "I am dressed in my riding suit, waiting for Father….I am going to try out Art Johnson's horse this morning, as he wants to sell it." Only when arthritis disabled her so she could not hold onto a horse's reins did Edith give up riding. It was one of the few things she noted regretting in old age.

Chuck remembered family parties as especially fun times. "Family gatherings…were many and large. Father had a sense of humor——he had to with all the children around. He used to squirt watermelon seeds [through his teeth] during the season, much to mother's consternation. Jokes of one type or another were constant, and Father would upset the teller by starting to laugh ahead of time, as he said, 'because I knew it was going to be so funny, I wouldn't have time to laugh enough afterwards.'"

Part of family life for Edith was making sure her children attended Sunday school, and when they had graduated from it, church. Each child was confirmed in the Episcopal church. Chuck had sufficient interest in religion to volunteer as a Sunday school teacher in his early teens. Once, his years of church-going with the family paid off in an unexpected way. At Hill School in Pottstown, Pennsylvania, he was elected president of the YMCA and asked to give a speech accepting the honor. He spent hours preparing a written text, but when he looked into the eyes of his audience, he grew terrified and his hands shook so violently he couldn't read his notes. As he described it, "I simply recited the Lord's Prayer and sat down. I think this first speech was better than any I have made since."

Young Edith was mortified on Sundays, sitting next to Dorothy at church, because Dorothy couldn't sing properly——she was loud and off key. Much later young Edith told her son how she felt cheated of some of her childhood, because she was the one child who was called on most often to tend Dorothy. Being a girl, and closest to Dorothy in age, she often got the caregiver job.

All the children were deprived of some attention their mother would naturally have given them if Dorothy hadn't needed her so much. But they benefited too. By watching their mother care for her afflicted child, they learned compassion for the unfortunate.

Esther got an extra bonus, since she learned to read when only four by sitting beside Dorothy when Edith patiently, with a sweet spirit, worked at teaching Dorothy to read, repeating over and over the sounds of the letters and words. For Esther it was a game she could play beside her dear mother, and without really understanding how it happened, Esther discovered she could read.

Edith liked to teach her children. According to Mayo, "She was constantly teaching [the children] something in a very lovely subtle way....Her friends always said how focused she was. It did not matter to whom she spoke – one of her children, one of the maids, the gardener, or an old man down the street – [at that moment, this] was the most important person in her life....Granny made everyone's life more palatable....She would often reach over while talking, and hold the person's hand, or touch them lightly on the shoulder...to let them know – I am here....I realize this was a special gift of hers."

Like her mother Jane Twentyman Graham, Edith continued nursing people, on an informal basis, her whole life. A nearby doctor, Dr. Dickson, esteemed her skills so much that he would sometimes come at night and waken her, if he had a problem with a sick person he couldn't handle by himself.

"She helped so many people," said her daughter Louise.

In later life Louise described growing up at Mayowood. "There was always a great deal of humor.... Everyone was fun....Life [for us children] was fairly regimented between the kitchen, the help, and the big play yard....Always lots of people at the house, people talking and walking around. They dressed for dinner, so it took time to be in early enough to clean up. The bells called us."

For Edith, the most important part of life in the Big House was her relationship with Charlie. According to her granddaughter Mayo, "They kissed often in front of the children and more often than not, touched in passing....Their affection was constant and open....It was actually fun to watch. Sometimes sitting at the table,...[the children] would catch them winking at each other. When she was long gone from the house...[my mother] carried that little picture of them winking and smiling at one another."

When Dr. Charlie came home from the Clinic each night, he would stand at the foot of the big entrance

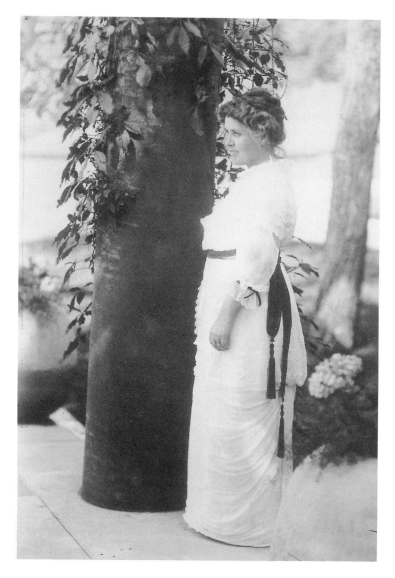

stairway, and before going up, purse his lips and make a certain whistle, which meant, "Edith! I'm home! Where are you?"

Soon from somewhere deep in the house, an answering whistle would come. Charlie would climb the stairs, and Edith would come to him. They would hug and kiss, and then, for a few minutes, sit together on the top step, softly whispering about the day. For this brief time, the children knew to leave them alone.

Mayo told of a day when her mother wanted to go out onto the patio to talk to her parents, but hesitated. "It was a beautiful morning," Mayo wrote, "and they sat out there in the sun, almost knee to knee. Mother noticed that Granddaddy held both of Granny's hands and was speaking softly. His face was about five inches from hers. They were leaning forward and intent and very dear. She stood by the unopened door watching and then left before they could catch her. She didn't wish to invade their moment."

Chapter 6

THE CHILDREN AND THE CLINIC MATURE

In September, 1913, at the age of 15, Chuck returned to his preparatory school, Hill School in Pennsylvania, and Joe accompanied him for the first time. Joe turned eleven on August 31; he was young to be leaving home, especially a home as interesting as Mayowood. Ever since he was a toddler, Joe had struck other people with his unusual exuberance and love of life. His brother later described him as "such a laughing man" and said, "He enjoyed life more than any[one] I ever knew. His style was to savor, his existence rollicking."

Unfortunately, Dr. Chuck said, Joe had another quality besides his free spirit: "his ill-starred fate to be caught in every wrongdoing." Joe's second year at Hill School, he was caught in some mischief and expelled, which greatly upset Edith and Dr. Charlie. They sent him on to Gilman Country School in Baltimore, Maryland, where, Dr. Chuck said, "mysteriously, he remained until graduation."

Edith and Dr. Charlie had decided to give their children educational advantages they themselves had lacked; instead of small town Rochester high schools, they preferred Eastern schools for their children.

Edith later told her granddaughter Mayo, "When the mind is opened and stretched by something new, it can never go back to where it was." Mayo saw this belief play out in her grandparents: "I think that is why they were so good and precious and loving and constantly growing."

The next year —1914 — was a year to stretch Edith. On March 6, the new Mayo Clinic Building was formally opened with receptions for about 1,600 people. It stood on the site of the house in which Dr. Charlie had been born. Now the various functions of the Clinic — diagnosis, consultation, surgery, and research — came under one roof, making this building the first in the world designed for the "integrated group practice of medicine," according to the Mayo Foundation. It was at this time the practice became officially known as "the Mayo Clinic."

Almost two years were required for the building's planning and construction, much of the planning done by Dr. Plummer, who designed for it the first telephone intercom system used in an American medical clinic. He also created an ingenious conveyor belt system for moving a patient's case history to the various doctors who wished to see it. In five floors were gathered business offices, examining rooms, x-ray cubicles and dark rooms, clinical laboratories, a big library, assembly hall, a pathologic museum, art studio, workshops for instrument-makers, and experimental laboratories with exercise areas for animals. It was a big step forward for the Clinic.

The reason for building the Mayo Clinic Building was, in Dr. Will's words, "to furnish a permanent house wherein scientific investigation can be made into the cause of the diseases which afflict mankind, and wherein every effort shall be made to cure the sick and the suffering." When it was first planned, the Drs. Mayo believed this structure would be sufficient for their practice for a long time and its use would be "permanent." But they didn't reckon on the amazing growth of their practice. In 1912, when the building was dedicated, Mayo patients numbered 15,000 people; by 1919, they numbered 60,000. In seven years the building was already inadequate.

On May 13, 1914, Edith and Dr. Charlie were saddened by the death of Edith's father, Joseph Graham, Senior, who passed away peacefully at the age of 91.

In June, July, and August, Edith accompanied Dr. Charlie on a trip to Europe with three Boston doctors. She left home alone by train on June 24, having said goodby to the children at Mayowood, "as it seemed it would be easier there than at station," she confided to her travel journal. Two days later, she met Charlie in New York City at 9:30 in the morning, shopped all day, and in the evening went to the Winter Garden with Charlie and Dr. Haggard, where "we saw a wonderful display of pretty faces and legs, particularly the latter."

The trip across the Atlantic by ship was restful and pleasant, except for some alarming news. At sea, one day out of New York, a report came that an assassin from Bosnia shot and killed Archduke Francis

Ferdinand, heir to the Austria-Hungarian throne, and his wife Sophie. (She had stepped in front of her husband to protect him.) Talk of impending war met Edith and Dr. Charlie wherever they traveled, casting an ominous pall over their journey.

They visited Germany, Denmark, Sweden, Norway, Holland and England, so that Charlie and the other doctors could meet European surgeons. Edith liked Sweden. "The [Baltic] Sea is beautiful, with many little rocky, wooded islands. The day perfect with best of company," she observed in her journal. As they neared Stockholm she noticed "a fine harbor, with high bluffs on all sides. Bathers in profusion abounded, without clothes and unembarrassed." In Stockholm, they went through the Royal Palace, which Edith described as "very much like other R.P.'s – big, cold, uncomfortable, formal, filled with ugly portraits of old queens and kings. Glad I do not happen to belong to the royal family of S."

In Norway, Edith observed near Bergen "the grandest scenery I have ever seen....We had a splendid drive, so we just enjoyed every moment. It is quite impossible to describe——-wonderful green mountains with lovely silver streams and dashing torrents...wonderful, wonderful." After spending Charlie's 49th birthday July 19 climbing a Norwegian mountain, with the help of some horses, Edith wrote, "It has been a day full of scenery such as I never hope to see equaled."

They traveled to London on July 26. There Dr. Charlie was elected president of the Clinical Congress of Surgeons of North America, and he delivered a paper accepting the position. World War I officially began on July 28. On July 31, at an elegant dinner party, Edith noted a "good deal of talk and worry about the war. England liable to be drawn into it. Germany after Russia. It means getting all Europe into a dreadful mix-up. Much fear that our boat Mauretania may not sail....A real excitement in the air of London. A great many worried Americans!"

The Mauretania did sail from Liverpool on August 1st. The next night Edith noted "still a little undercurrent of fear our ship may be recalled," but she enjoyed dancing in the evening. On August 4 and 5, persons on the ship reported sighting German cruisers, so "canvases were nailed up at doors to keep the lights from showing." Edith found this "very exciting, especially in daytime and no fog—-not so funny at night."

The ship stopped abruptly at 2 a.m. the morning of August 6, because German cruisers were sighted in the area. It diverted course and sailed to Halifax, Nova Scotia, where the anchor was let down for awhile, but eventually it sailed on to New York City. Edith and Dr. Charlie made their way home to Minnesota and a mighty welcome from their children.

Dr. Charlie's mother, Louise Abigail Wright Mayo, died on July 15, 1915. She had fallen and broken her hip one night, when she slipped off the step of her home while going outside to call her cat. Confined to bed and then to a wheelchair, she failed to rally and passed away at the age of 89. One year earlier, to a magazine interviewer Mrs. Mayo revealed the source of her strength in hard times: "If one doesn't give in under calamity, but just says, 'I'm going to be useful until I drop,' it helps a lot, my dear." Both Edith and Charlie grieved her loss; she had been a close friend to them and the children. Charlie's sense of humor and love of people, some said, came from his mother.

Edith's delight in helping people came from her own mother; one form it took was finding parents for homeless babies. One day in late 1915, Edith invited her chauffeur, Carlos Ellis, and his wife, Lenora Stedman Ellis, who were childless, to dinner at the Big House. When everyone had finished eating, Edith said, "Come on upstairs. I have something to show you."

In an upstairs bedroom lay a baby girl, asleep in a cradle. "She is for you," Edith said. "You may take her home."

Carlos and Lenora were overjoyed to adopt the baby. They named her "Esther," probably in honor of Edith's youngest child.

Another form of good deed which Edith enjoyed was

corresponding with people, not only her friends and family, but former Mayo Clinic patients as well. During World War I she wrote frequently to Mr. and Mrs. Herman Kloninger, whom she had met when they came to the Clinic for treatment. The couple was German and had been living in the United States, but sought refuge from anti-German sentiment here to live quietly in Budleigh Salterton, Devon, England. Her letters to them were long and full of maternal concern for their well being. She even forwarded a medical question from Mr. Kloninger to a Mayo Clinic doctor, who advised him from afar. Mrs. Kloninger mysteriously died during the war, and her husband wrote Edith to pour out his grief.

For Christmas of 1915, someone gave Chuck a journal so he could record the events of his life. He was 17, in his next-to-last year at Hill School, and the place still did not please him. His entries began on New Year's day. Home for Christmas break, he observed, "The worst thing about coming home is that one hates so bad to leave again."

On January 6, 1916, Chuck did "something most unusual for me. I got up at 6:30 and went down with Father to the hospital and saw a bunch of operations...a carcinoma of the breast, a bunch of goiters, and appendixes, etc." Dr. Charlie was attempting to do for his son what his own father had done for him——-initiate

him early into the mysteries of surgery. This particular day, Chuck enjoyed watching his father at work, but what he liked even better was watching the animals upstairs on the research floor. "Gosh, they had a peach of a monkey," he said.

The next day, January 7, Dr. Charlie took him again to the hospital. This was an important day in Chuck's life, for he decided "I am darned shure [sic] now that I would rather be a surgeon than any other profession that I can think of....Believe me but this is the life."

Chuck's visit home for spring break gives a small view of the activities in the Big House in 1916. On Sunday, April 2, he went to church with Mother and Dorothy. It was Esther's seventh birthday, so in the evening a family party drove into Rochester to see the play, "Cabiria." In addition to Edith, Dr. Charlie, and the children, two cousins went along, Kit Olin and Don Twentyman. The next evening Edith took a bunch of flowers down to Rochester to her brother, Dr. Kit, in celebration of his 60th birthday.

Two cousins stayed all night with Chuck and Joe the following Saturday night, Rodney Waldron and Don Twentyman again. Then, on Sunday, "a peach of a day," the family, including Dr. Charlie, rose early and all went to church.

"The sermon wasn't bad," Chuck said. In the evening Edith, her sister Margaret Twentyman, Dorothy, and Chuck went down to Rochester again to a concert in the

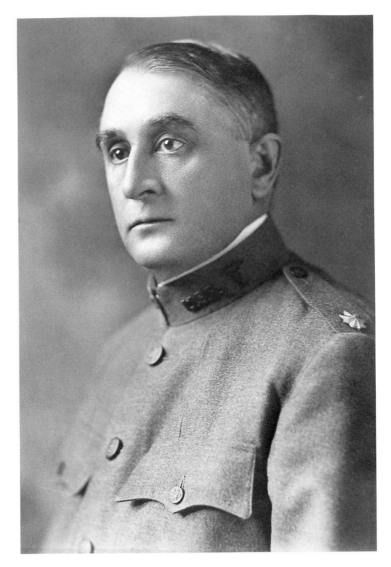

Methodist Church.

Chuck's vacation ended on Wednesday, April 12. Edith traveled along with Chuck and Joe to Chicago so she could see them safely on the overnight train to Philadelphia. She considered them old enough to negotiate the change of trains there. Chuck noted in his journal, "The train of sorrow left Philadelphia at 1:10 p.m. for Pottstown."

He continued the journal into June, where one of the last entries, on June 18, noted: "Father elected president of American Medical Association. Proud son." After completing his examinations at the Hill School, Chuck boarded the train for home and never again wrote in his journal. He was headed for Mayowood and summer and had better things to do.

On April 6, 1917, when America entered the world war, Dr. Charlie and Dr. Will were both made colonels in the Surgeon General's office. (They were promoted to brigadier generals four years later.) Renting an apartment in Washington, D.C., they rotated residences there for the rest of the war, spending six weeks in Washington, followed by six weeks in Rochester, so that one of them was always in attendance at the Clinic. Up to now, Dr. Charlie's schedule, though busy and punctuated by frequent separations from his family, had always allowed time for family and fun. Now it became a hectic life with unending work, which he was willing to endure because of devotion to his country.

The burden of caring for the family fell more heavily on Edith while Dr. Charlie was in Washington. The children had been taught from babyhood never to raise their voices against mother or father; the exception was Dorothy. Occasionally, she would stamp her foot and noisily complain to Edith about a grievance, especially if she felt another child had been allowed a favor she was denied. Only to Edith would Dorothy do this, because Edith listened patiently to her afflicted daughter and tried to pacify her. Dorothy knew no one else would pay the slightest bit of attention to her, so she didn't fuss at anyone else.

An example of the quiet way Edith liked to keep order is a story her daughter told. Louise had heard a member of the household staff describe an angry woman by saying she was "het up." So one day at dinner, speaking of an angry friend, Louise said, "She was all het up."

Immediately, Edith rose from the table and marched to her office, ordering Louise to come along. Inside, Edith closed the door and spoke with great seriousness to Louise. "You must never again use that expression," she said. "It can be taken in another way."

This was discipline enough. Louise never again used that phrase.

The stress of overwork in Washington and Rochester made Dr. Charlie vulnerable to illness; he contracted pneumonia while in Washington. Eventually, with rest, he recovered, since the type of pneumonia which sickened him was not a deadly type.

⸙

During these years Dr. Will and Dr. Charlie made three important decisions which affected the future of the Mayo Clinic, insuring its development into an institution which would thrive even without them. First, they turned the Mayo partnership into a corporation in 1915. Each of the partners, including Dr. Will and Dr. Charlie, signed a document in which he relinquished all rights to the partnership, agreeing to accept a salary arrangement and one year's salary as a parting settlement when he left the practice. Without such an agreement, any one partner's heirs could have sued the Clinic for a share of its total assets, if they chose, upon the death of the partner.

For Dr. Graham, signing was difficult, because it meant giving up a large amount of money which he had, in fact, helped earn. But he did sign.

Dr. Chuck said, "I've realized many times since what a masterful piece of forethought is represented by that agreement. It means that I and my children don't own the Clinic, or any part of it, so as a principal victim I am in a good position to say how much I admire it.

Without it, the Mayo Clinic would have been in fragments generations ago, pulled apart by the descendants of doctors."

The second decision Dr. Will and Dr. Charlie made was to give away all their accumulated joint fortune, $1,500,000, establishing with it the Mayo Foundation for Medical Education in conjunction with the University of Minnesota, which became the Mayo Graduate School of Medicine, the world's first graduate program training medical specialists. Edith approved this noble and sacrificial step.

As Dr. Will explained in a speech before the Minnesota legislature, this was done so that "'These dead shall not have died in vain.' That line explains why we want to do this thing. What better could we do than help young men become proficient in the profession so as to prevent needless death?"

The third important decision also required sacrifice from all the Clinic's former partners. All properties belonging to the Mayo Clinic, amounting to more than ten million dollars, were to be deeded away to the Mayo Foundation, removing all control of the Clinic from the Mayo family and partners. This was the final reorganizational move which created the Mayo Clinic as it is today. Again Dr. Kit was asked to sign away a fortune.

When Chuck Mayo returned home in December, 1918, from Princeton (where he had enrolled after Hill School), he walked into what he called "the family disaster that lasted through Christmas…and well into the following year." Dr. Graham refused to sign this second agreement. His reasons, according to Dr. Chuck, were, "He had endured stripping his descendants of most of their legacy, but this final disinheritance was too much."

Clapesattle attributed other motives to him. "Dr. Graham was too wholeheartedly a clinician to be able to appreciate his partners' efforts toward making research and education auxiliary functions of the Clinic. He had disapproved of the Foundation and its affiliation with the university, and when it came to underwriting that affiliation by assigning the assets of the partnership to [it], he refused to give his consent."

Edith was in the middle of the storm, pleading with Charlie to take Kit's part and dissuade Will from this idea. For once, she put the good of her brother before the good of the Clinic. According to Dr. Chuck, "Father kept quiet; he deemed it inadvisable to admit to Mother that every detail of the plan was as much his as Uncle Will's, and that he was in total agreement. Angry and bitter, Uncle Kit resigned." Both Drs. Mayo were, Chuck said, "desolated by his decision, but they didn't hesitate to accept his resignation. Mother was in tears for days."

In time, Kit Graham agreed with Dr. Will that the educational aim of the Clinic was as important as its treatment aim, and a reconciliation took place between the two men. Edith wrote Chuck at Princeton in May, 1921, "You will be glad to know that Uncle Will and Uncle Kit have become reconciled. I'll tell you about it when I see you. Uncle Will made the first advances in a very fine way."

When World War I ended, Dr. Charlie was again able to return to the work he loved best: surgery and teaching at the Mayo Clinic. On July 9, 1918, President Woodrow Wilson and the Congress presented to Dr. Charlie and Dr. Will "a Distinguished Service Medal...awarded to you...for exceptionally meritorious and conspicuous service."

By now, some of the children were becoming adults. When it was time for young Edith to leave for college, she told her parents she wanted to attend art school. But they were as ambitious for their daughters as for their sons.

Edith told her daughter, "No. You are going to college. You will be the first woman in the family to go to college and earn a degree." Four years later, Edith graduated from Vassar College, where she studied art and other subjects. She enjoyed painting all her life.

Louise was encouraged to develop her talents too. Edith and Dr. Charlie sent her to Miss Spence's Finishing School and the Art Student's League in New York City.

During the summers, when she was a teen, Louise worked as a medical artist at the Mayo Clinic, encouraged by her father, who also liked to draw. She said later, "Father...could sketch anything and would pick up every detail of his subject with his skilled hands. We would have great drawing contests with mother cheering in the background."

Disciplining the children was important to Edith. With them all, she used the same firm hand. When her daughters grew interested in boys, she was careful. A popular teen activity in Rochester on summer weekends was dancing parties. Edith allowed Louise to go, but not with a date. Instead, the chauffeur drove Louise to the parties and picked her up again. Fifty years later, Louise told an interviewer how embarrassed she was when she looked up from her dancing partner and saw the chauffeur standing in the door, ready to drive her home. She felt, "Mother was affecting my life too much and wasn't letting me live like others could live."

Edith expected her teenage children to keep a curfew too, and she was strict and consistent about enforcing it. For Louise in her teens, the curfew was 11 p.m. If some circumstance kept Louise out later, she knew what to expect: her mother would be sitting on a chair at the top of the broad flight of stairs in the entranceway to the Big House, waiting. When Louise entered, she would rise

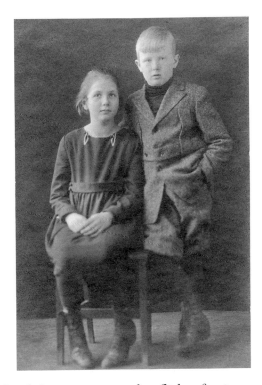

without a word and disappear up another flight of stairs into the big southwest bedroom she shared with Dr. Charlie. That night, Louise would have no good night kiss. It was a very effective discipline method.

On April 2, 1920, Edith's youngest child, Esther, celebrated her eleventh birthday. About this time, she and Louise began begging their mother to adopt a baby. Several years earlier Edith and Dr. Charlie had brought a foster child into the family, a little eighteen-month boy named John Nelson, whom they saved from being sent to an orphanage when his mother's family could care for him no longer. He turned nine on February 19, so he couldn't satisfy the girls' desires for a baby. Edith was open to her daughters' request – with John Nelson and a new baby, she would be able to rear eight children after all, replacing the two girls who had died, Margaret and Rachel.

So Edith took Esther and Louise into Rochester, to a home for unwanted babies which Edith helped support. Finding homes for babies was important to Edith throughout her life. In her volunteer efforts on the babies' behalf, she was working as Dr. Charlie's partner. He opposed abortion as a method of birth control and believed finding loving adoptive parents for unwanted babies was a far better option. Once, when a woman insisted on an abortion, he told her, with heavy irony, "You go ahead and have the baby, and after it is born, you and I will take it out to the barn and chop it to pieces."

The home for babies where Edith took Esther and Louise was a place she loved to visit. Susie Graham, Edith's widowed sister-in-law, ran the home. Besides her own eight children, Susie cared for as many as eight homeless babies at a time, as well as unmarried, pregnant girls. Mayo described the atmosphere of Susie's house: "Aunt Susie was round and kissy....She always had loads of white laundry flying on the lines and plenty of cookies and wonderful cornbread cooked in round tin cans. It was a very busy place...and crowded with activity that always gave Aunt Susie that little ruffled look....[Granny] and Aunt Susie were very close. Granny said how she loved to go down there... for it reminded her of Grahamholm. Granny was always trying to find parents for Aunt Susie's babies."

It must have given Edith satisfaction on this day when she herself volunteered to become a mother for one of Susie's adoptable infants.

"Go ahead and pick out a baby," Edith told her daughters.

In less than five minutes, Esther chose a lovely little dark-haired girl with expressive brown eyes, who responded to her with big grins. Edith told Esther this was an excellent decision. Then she added, "Many people looking for a baby would find it easy to choose that precious little girl."

In another crib was a baby who might never be chosen. She had blonde hair and pretty blue eyes, but her skin was badly blotched with eczema. She looked like she needed a home. Edith persuaded Esther and Louise that this little girl was the right one for them; they

brought her home; Edith and Dr. Charlie adopted her.

The baby was named Marilynn, but everyone called her Sally. Born just two days after Esther's eleventh birthday, on April 4, 1920, Sally needed lots of care. Even though Edith was already 53 years old, she rose at 5:30 every morning to give the child her morning feeding.

Nine years later, Edith described Sally in a letter to Esther, who was away from home at an Italian finishing school. "Sally just came in and glanced over my shoulder and read 'Dearest of Esthers,' then kissed and hugged me and said, 'I am the dearest of Sallys, aren't I?' and then, 'I love Esther; she is comical, isn't she?' and went out to her breakfast. School opens for her today, and I think she is not sorry, for I have made her practice her piano every day and do at least an hour in arithmetic, besides some work in language....I can see that child develop from day to day, and if nothing happens to her, she is going to be a credit to us."

Edith and Dr. Charlie raised both John Nelson and Sally to adulthood. John graduated from college with a degree in engineering and became a mining engineer. He married and was the father of four children during Edith's lifetime, including a son named "Joseph Graham Nelson." Edith corresponded with her foster son each week from the time he went away to boarding school in his early teens until her death.

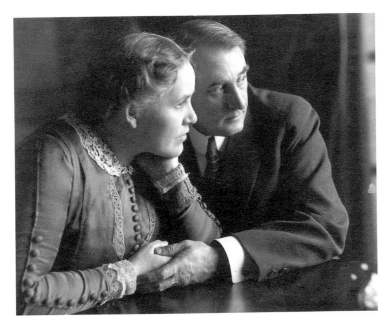

Sally attended Northwestern University in Evanston, Illinois. She helped America fight in World War II as a "W.A.C." in the Women's Army Corps. On August 6, 1943, eleven days after Edith died, Sally married Lieutenant Ralph S. Mason in a small family wedding ceremony at Mayowood. Edith had met the bridegroom and liked him. She had helped as much as she could in Sally's decisions about flowers, the wedding gown, and so on. Like her sister Esther, Sally carried a small prayer book interlaced with ribbons as she exchanged vows with her husband. She was beautiful in her full length silk gown, the deep V neckline edged with lace. She wore a fingertip chapel veil of lace. Mayo said: "Lt. Mason and Sally wore their uniforms to the reception and stood proudly straight in them. Mother [Louise Mayo Trenholm] gave the reception for them at Ivy Cottage. I was impressed, for they looked so important and American....This wedding was such a sign of the times. Granny had died not too many days before, and there was still a sadness in the air."

In 1921, another wedding brought Edith joy. Phoebe Mayo, who had been born to Dr. Will and Hattie two days after Dorothy's birth, married Dr. Waltman Walters February 5 in a beautiful wedding ceremony.

For Dr. Charlie and Edith, an even bigger event came on Tuesday, June 12, 1923 – the wedding of Edith, the first of their children to marry. The groom was Dr. Fred Wharton Rankin from Mooresville, North Carolina. He had come to the Clinic as a fellow in surgery. During World War I, he served as surgeon in France at Base Hospital No. 26, called "the Mayo unit" because it was partly funded by the Mayo brothers and one-third of its personnel came from the Clinic. Then following the war, he returned to the Clinic to

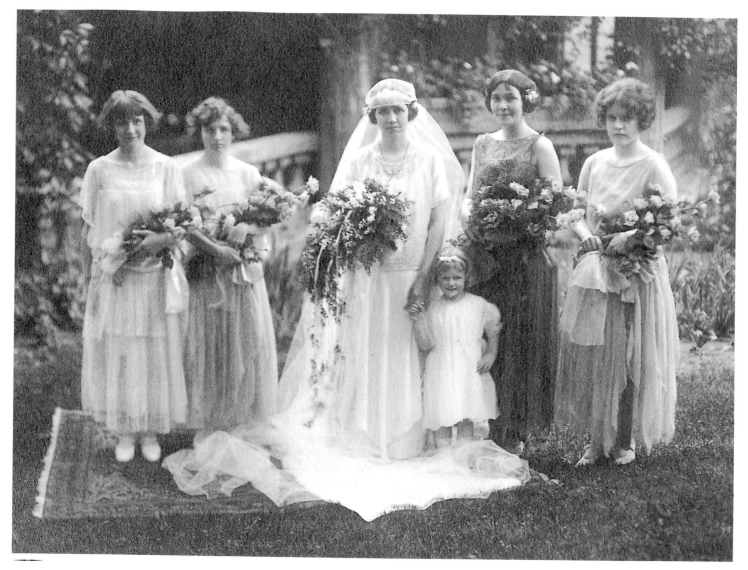

complete his surgical training. This is when he and young Edith courted and fell in love.

During the year after she graduated from Vassar in June, 1922, Edith enjoyed living at home. She returned to Rochester a glamourous 21-year-old, driving a four-door Cadillac Phaeton which her parents gave as her graduation present. "If I hadn't been promised an automobile when I got through college, I don't think I ever would have gotten through," she said later. "I used to let it purr gently down Broadway and show people how slowly I could go. The top, of course, came down, and I kept it down most of the time." Young Edith at this time studied to be a nurse like her mother and in three months earned her cap and pin. Then she decided, instead of continuing nursing, to marry Dr. Fred.

According to the *Rochester Daily Bulletin*, their wedding was "one of the most beautiful home weddings of the season." The living room of the Big House was decorated in pink roses, white lilies and green canterbury bells, setting a color theme which was continued in the wedding supper decor. Outside in the courtyard, supper was served to 160 guests. Planning and preparing for the wedding had been an exciting activity for both Ediths, mother and daughter, for months before the event.

Young Edith chose her sisters, Dorothy, Louise and Esther as bridesmaids, and her three-year-old sister Sally as flower girl. The wedding march was played on the organ by a friend of the groom, Dr. Phillip Hench, accompanied by 12-year-old Johnny Nelson. (Dr. Hench much later – in 1950 – won the Nobel Prize with Dr. Edward C. Kendall for their work discovering cortisone.) At the end of the living room, before an improvised altar, the Reverend Arthur H. Wurtele, rector of Calvary Episcopal Church, performed the traditional wedding ceremony.

Edith and Dr. Fred honeymooned in Minneapolis and then drove Edith's Cadillac to their new home in Louisville, Kentucky, where Dr. Rankin was professor of surgery at the University of Louisville and also in charge of surgery at Louisville City Hospital. Soon, because of this marriage, another chapter in Edith's life developed – grandmotherhood.

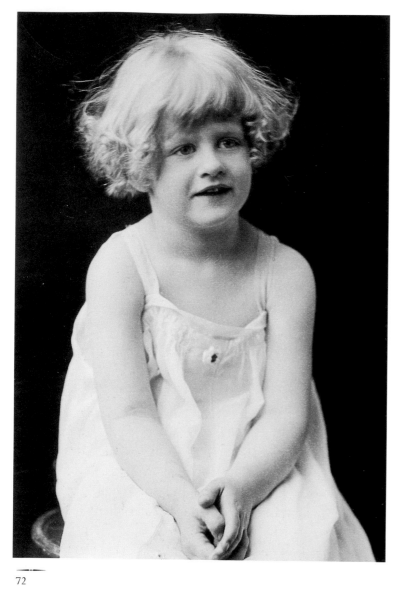

Sally Mayo in 1924

Photo courtesy of Mayo Kooiman

Chapter 7

GRANDMOTHERHOOD

By the time she was 57, Edith was beginning to look like a grandmother. She was now "a little bit round," according to her granddaughter Mayo. Her long straight hair, turned from dark brown to white, she wore coiled back from her face. It shone like a halo when the light was behind her. She was still beautiful. Her large, expressive brown eyes were bright, and, almost always, her lips curled in a small smile, as if she were enjoying a secret joke.

Her grandson Charles Rankin described her as "truly a beautiful woman to my small mind. She had the most wonderful smile, bright eyes, enthusiastic voice. You know another memory I have? Her perfume. Granny always pleasured me just to sit on her lap."

Edith was afflicted by arthritis, especially in her hands. The joints were swollen, and bumps were beginning to form on the knuckles. Mayo said, "She hated her hands, which hurt big time." Shaking hands became a form of torture for Edith – she was sometimes required to shake 60 to 100 hands at a time. So she worked out a way to spare herself pain. When a person extended his hand to her, she quickly slid her hand into his, snugly as possible slipping the hollow between her thumb and forefinger into the hollow between his. If she could slide her hand into his fast enough, before he began squeezing her hand, she wouldn't be hurt.

In a winter letter to her daughter Esther, Edith mentioned her arthritis. "We have really had wild weather since Friday, but I like it if I don't have to get out in it too much. I loved facing the elements long ago, but the cold makes my arthritis more painful, so I am more or less 'an Edith sit-by-the-fire' now."

Two weeks after her 57th birthday (in 1924), the first of Edith's 21 grandchildren was born. The baby was due about March 15; young Edith returned to Rochester in mid-February to prepare for the birth, with Dr. Fred planning to come later, just in time. The night of February 26, labor pains woke young Edith. She hurried into her parents' bedroom with the news.

"I guess I'm having some trouble here," she said.

Dr. Charlie, still half asleep, responded, "You can't! – for another two weeks!"

Reasonably, Edith the soon-to-be-grandmother said, "Now, Charlie, be calm. Just call the hospital. I think we have to go to the hospital – This is it!"

At noon the next day the baby arrived. He was named Fred Wharton Rankin, Jr., after his father, and nicknamed "Buck." Because the baby soon left for Louisville, Kentucky, with his parents, the new "Granny" had to be satisfied with loving him from afar.

Of course, her other children still required attention. Sally, who was not yet four, spent all of her time at home. The other young children, John, Esther and Louise, all attended boarding schools and were always

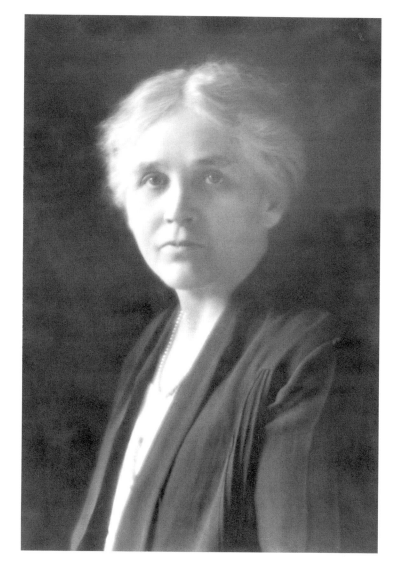

home for vacations and summers. Chuck and Joe were
in medical school, Chuck at the University of
Pennsylvania, Joe at the University of Iowa. Dorothy,
now 27, still attended school, a boarding school in
Winona, Minnesota, run by the Sisters of Saint Francis,
the same teaching order of nuns who had built St.
Mary's Hospital back in 1889.

On April 23, 1924, Dorothy wrote her mother from
school:

"Dear Mother,

*...I am having a good time with the sisters and the girls. I
went for work today and played croquet with the girls after
dinner....I am reading a book....I am doing what you told me
to do.*

With love,
Dorothy Mayo."

Edith's life was as busy as ever. She traveled
frequently; in late spring of 1925 she and Louise
accompanied Dr. Charlie on another trip to Europe.
(About this time Charlie's friend Dr. Haggard referred
to him and Dr. Will as "the surgical travelers of the
world.") Because the Doctors Mayo were friends with
many doctors, they were often chosen to be leaders
when doctors toured surgical centers in Europe for

postgraduate study. So it was on this trip. Dr. Charlie was in charge of more than 100 surgeons. He supervised their travel in Great Britain, France and Austria, presided at discussion groups following clinics, and served as their spokesman at all social functions. The days were full. Dr. Charlie met Madame Curie, the Duke of York, and King George of England and spoke with them in the name of the other doctors. He received honorary degrees at the University of Edinburgh, Scotland, and at Queen's University in Belfast, Ireland, giving speeches for these events. Dr. Charlie arrived home exhausted. When strokes weakened him five years later, Dr. Will said he believed this trip was partly the cause.

At Mayowood, Edith continued as an "unflappable" hostess, according to Dr. Chuck, "even in the face of Father's impulsive tendency to invite visiting doctors and their entire families to stay at Mayowood for as long as they liked." Once Dr. Charlie phoned Edith to tell her that 100 medical librarians had visited the Clinic and were on their way to Mayowood at his invitation. "Would she show them around?" Of course she did.

Edith especially enjoyed parties for friends and family. When the children came home from boarding school, she planned big parties for them. Daughter Edith later said, "All the young folks [of Rochester] always used to love to come out to Mayowood." About three times a year, Edith would hold a big party for one or more of her children, often a costume party or formal ball. Young Edith remembered a party in the ballroom with the Harold Cook orchestra providing music. Everyone wore evening clothes, and this particular summer evening, watermelon was served out on the lawn. "You were careful not to spill on your ballgown," she said.

Nine of Edith's siblings were still alive in 1925, and she had 40 living nieces and nephews, many of them married with children, and most of them living near Rochester. They were frequent guests at her house. She wrote Chuck about a party she gave that year with 75 guests, dressed in clothes of the 1870's. Tables were laid for them in the gallery and two dining rooms; a dinner of "peanuts (salted, prepared at home)," ham, scalloped potatoes, rutabagas, cucumber pickles, slaw, hot biscuits with honey and butter, and coffee was served, with pumpkin pie, cheese, and "big, soft cookies with a raisin in the center of each" for dessert.

Then the party was moved to the ballroom for dancing. Edith had engaged a fiddler, who was accompanied by Uncle Kit and Aunt Blanche, Kit's wife. The program began with "a Grand March, then…a few old-fashioned waltzes scattered through the evening, the old Sour Kraut, Virginia Reel, three-step, polkas, heel and toe, two Schottisches, two quadrilles and end[ed] up with Home Sweet Home." For the best dancers, Edith had purchased "marvellous prizes." She also provided tables with cards for people too tired to dance. Arthritis in her hands didn't keep Edith off the dance floor.

Dr. Chuck received another letter from his mother, whom he called "that prodigious woman," describing how she had served "dinner for 53 last night, and had the Magazine Club out today, 100 strong, and had a good time. Have Auntie Trude's club tomorrow." [Auntie Trude was Gertrude Mayo Berkman, Dr. Charlie's older sister, a much loved member of the family.]

One day Dorothy told her mother she didn't want to go to school anymore. Her sister Edith wasn't going to school, and, Dorothy pointed out, she was older than Edith. "I want to work," Dorothy said.

As usual, Edith tried to accommodate her daughter. She asked the nursing nuns at St. Mary's Hospital if they would create a job for Dorothy; Edith wanted to provide money for wages. They obliged and Dorothy began carrying trays and rolling bandages for a wage of 30 dollars a month. There was a problem, though, because Dorothy was, in her sister Louise's words, "inclined to talk quite a bit." The nuns eventually moved her to the children's floor of the hospital, where she was happiest, because she was mentally like a child herself.

One day Dorothy arrived home from work and told her mother, "I'm striking. If this goes through, I'll get a dollar more a month." Her salary was raised from $30 to $31.

On New Year's Day, 1926, Edith's second grandchild was born and named for her, Edith Graham Rankin. So eager was Edith to receive this little one into the family, she traveled for the birth to Lexington, Kentucky (where the Rankins had relocated). The baby was originally expected about Thanksgiving; Edith came then. By January first, when the baby finally arrived, Edith was very anxious to return to Mayowood and Dr. Charlie. Never before had she been away from him at Christmastime in all the 33 years of their marriage. Fondly, Edith congratulated her daughter and son-in-law, kissed the baby and her big brother, and headed straight home.

Little Edith was the second child of daughter Edith and Dr. Rankin, a little sister for Buck. To distinguish her from her mother and grandmother, the family always called her "Missey." The baby, like her mother, looked like Granny.

Six months after Missey's birth, Edith was overjoyed when the Rankin family returned to Rochester. Dr. Rankin joined the Mayo Clinic as head of a section of surgery and also associate professor of surgery in the Mayo Foundation. He and his family moved into "White Gables," a house on Mayowood Road across from two large stone barns and a big field.

Being a grandmother was delightful for Edith, but being a mother still posed its problems. Joe had dropped out of Princeton University, but by summer, 1926, he seemed to be doing well at the University of Iowa. Dr. Chuck explained, "Joe's progress through school was a saga, punctuated by Mother pleading with deans to give him another chance....He had no luck in getting away with anything."

Esther was a problem too. After finishing at the Laurel School in Cleveland, Ohio, Esther still needed more math training before she could qualify for college. She had somehow slipped through school without taking algebra. Edith and Dr. Charlie decided an elite eastern boarding school, the Choate School in Brookline, Massachusetts, was the right place to help her complete high school work. As with Chuck and Joe, Esther resisted going so far from home. Now 17, Esther was so upset she wrote to her parents, protesting, and also to her brother Chuck:

"Dearest Chuck,

"The family has at last resorted to force, and that means I have to go to that vile Choate school. Makes me simply furious because I loathe it and every one connected with it, and my entire summer has been ruined. Furthermore, I've lost my only good friend and will probably be more miserable next year than I already anticipate, and if I am, I shall probably die."

Edith and Dr. Charlie concluded that Esther was overreacting, in the manner of some teens. She was, at this time, given to theatrical exaggeration and somewhat insecure about her intellectual abilities; she wore lenseless glasses frames to make herself look smarter. The reasons Esther gave for disliking Choate were not sufficient to convince her parents: "It's one of those ungodly forsaken places where you're asked to bring two hats – both simple – one for church and one for street wear, an umbrella, rubber overshoes and long sleeved, high necked nighties. I'm just sick and I've cried three days straight."

During Esther's year in Massachusetts, Edith wrote her faithfully, once a week or more often. Her letters were full of good advice. For instance, Edith wrote her daughter: "I'm tickled to pieces with your work in philosophy and Browning – better send your paper on to me. I haven't read Galahad, but I did read Helen of Troy. Very modern indeed, but unusual and interesting in a way. I hardly think you'll enjoy it. It lacks cleanliness, I think....They should not let obscene literature through the mails. [Rabbi Wise] considered both Galahad and Helen of Troy obscene literature. Perhaps that is carrying it too far, but I wish you would read more biography and history and books that are uplifting, including Will Rogers."

The next year, 1927, was full of events – a death and two weddings. Just past Edith's sixtieth birthday, her sister Margaret Graham Twentyman died of cancer on March 8, at the age of 64. It was an early death for a Graham. Margaret spent her last four months in the

Big House in a bedroom separated by a bathroom from another bedroom, where her sister Dinah, suffering from pernicious anemia and diabetes, was staying. Edith helped nurse both sisters.

Writing to her brother Dr. Kit, Edith spoke of her feelings for Margaret: "We certainly loved her, didn't we?…Kit, there were so many gifts that came from Grahamholm. We were so blessed. Every time you smile I am able to see each member of my family. I love you deeply and constantly pray for you….and precious, lovable and laughable Maggie."

Edith's son Joe was the first son to marry, but Chuck was the first to propose to his future bride. In January, Chuck and Alice Varney Plank from Philadelphia, Pennsylvania, became engaged, planning to wed in June when Chuck finished his internship at Robert Packer Hospital in Sayre, Pennsylvania. Joe, 24 and four years younger than Chuck, was in his final year of medical school with his internship still to serve. But he was in love with Ruth Rakowsky, a beautiful 18-year-old girl who was born in Duluth, Minnesota, and reared in Joplin, Missouri. (They met when Ruth was a patient at the Clinic, seeking the explanation of symptoms which turned out to be diabetes.) When Joe heard the news of his older brother's engagement, he impetuously decided to propose to Ruth and marry her, also in June.

Edith was deeply upset when the letter came from Joe telling of this plan. She assumed that Joe was not planning to complete his medical preparation and would have to work as something other than a doctor. Since Dr. Charlie was out of town when Joe's letter came, she answered it herself the same day she received it, January 14, 1927:

"*My dear son,*

"*It is ten o'clock p.m., but I am going to chat awhile with you before going to bed, as your letter has more or less upset me, and depressed me, and I must tell you what I think, regardless of your feelings.…*

"*[Your father] is very much pleased with [Ruth's] improvement and the way her care is managed by her mother and herself. So far as marrying is concerned, he thinks she should have more time in which to perfect herself as far as possible. She will always have to…care for her health, of course, and I am sure neither of you will ever regret considering her health first, and your immediate happiness second.*

"*…If you do consider what is for her good, putting your own desires out of the question entirely, it will be the first sacrifice of your life, and will be proof to us that your love for Ruth is the enduring kind, which is the only sort that grows better with the passing years. Ruth is a beautiful girl with heaps of good sense, but she is young and can afford to give her parents another year of herself.…And if your love cannot endure the strain of a few months waiting and working and sacrifice for her — beware — it's passion and not love that controls you. I hate that word, which shouldn't get mixed up with love — they* *are not even second cousins.*

"...Look at your record at Hill, Gilman and Princeton — you could have been more than an average student if you had tried just a little bit — if you could have sacrificed your self, what you thought your pleasures, your appetite, to please us....Anyway, we stood by you through thick and thin, feeling sure that somehow, some way, the good in you would win out. And the last two years...have been so much better, we have taken heart mightily.

"There is so much that is sweet and lovable about you. You have somehow been able to slip and slide out of everything distasteful — to avoid all responsibility, which we have ever tried to make you understand was yours....Now we have come to this biggest thing in your life. Are you going to start out on that journey all unprepared and choose another easier way of making a living? We can't have any but first class doctors in the family. You have every quality to make our kind but stick-to-itiveness, which you must cultivate, my dear.

"You have Ruth to win. You have her love — earn her respect and the respect and admiration of everyone by taking the next year and a half to study, work, and conquer yourself. You will always be glad for it, and you have your whole life ahead of you. And while you will be doing it for her, it will make us feel happy, too.

"You will never know, unless sometime you have a 'Joe' of your own, how much your Father and I have loved you, do love you."

Several days later Louise wrote Chuck, describing their future sister-in-law: Ruth "is terribly attractive. Rather exotic looking. Only 18, but quite mature....She looks sophisticated and blase, but isn't the

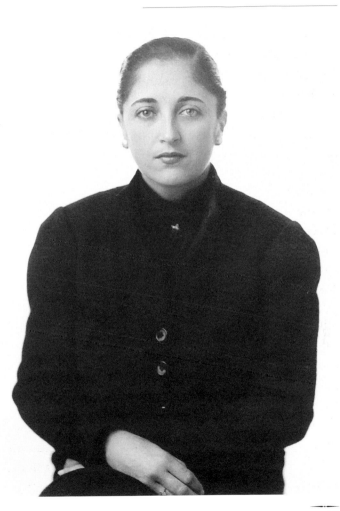

Ruth Rakowski, who married Dr. Joe Mayo in 1927

Photo courtesy of Mayo Kooiman

least bit – in fact, is very natural. Her skin is very dark, making her look tanned all the time. Her eyes are green with heavy, dark, long eyelashes. Her cheeks and lips are naturally quite vivid, which contrasts with everything and makes her stunning. She's as tall as Joe and large boned, very muscular and healthy looking….Ruth is, I think, too easy with Joe. She thinks everything he does is cute. Maybe it's because she's young."

By May the question of when Joe and Ruth would marry was settled, – in June, just as he originally intended – and Edith resigned herself to it. Joe was completing his medical studies creditably at the University of Iowa. Better yet, he had secured an internship at Scott and White Hospital in Temple, Texas, and Mrs. A.C. Scott was making arrangements for Ruth and Joe's home in Temple after their marriage. Edith wrote her younger son on May 6,
"Dearest Joseph,

"I am enclosing a letter from Mrs. Scott which I know will set your mind at rest. I, too, feel relieved and so will Ruth, so send it on to her."

Ruth's father and mother had just visited at Mayowood, and Edith wrote, *"The more I see and know of the Rakowskys, the better I like them. In fact, I wouldn't change one of them the least little bit. I feel a very motherly love for dear Ruth, and I am sure you and she will be very very happy. Be tender and patient with her always, and love her unselfishly. I am sure you will, as the Mayos and Grahams are all one woman men and true to the end, and you can be no exception with such a girl as Ruth to love and be loved by."*

And so, the first Mayo wedding of the year, on Saturday, June 11, was between Joe and Ruth. She had, by this time, turned 19. The wedding ceremony took place at 10 a.m. in the large living room of the bride's parents' home in Joplin. According to the *Rochester Post Bulletin*, Ruth wore "a smart gown of white organdie and old lace with a touch of white satin." Her veil was long and made of rare lace. In her arms she carried a bouquet of roses, orange blossoms and lilacs. Janis was her sister's maid of honor, and Dr. Fred Rankin served as best man for Joe, since Chuck was in the last week of his internship and planning his own wedding and therefore couldn't make the trip from Philadelphia to Missouri. Ruth's brother Russell Rakowsky was an usher.

Writing from home to Chuck a week later, Edith described the wedding. Dr. Fred and Edith Rankin, John Nelson, Dr. Charlie and Edith had traveled to Missouri for the event which "was small (only 22 counting minister, groom, bride, musicians and all), but it was perfect to the least detail….Flowers [were] in profusion, good music, pretty gowns and bridesmaids, and Ruth looked like a gypsy princess, simply radiant. They had the Episcopal service, which was very dignified and solemn, and both Joe and Ruth responded in well modulated tones."

After the wedding, Joe and Ruth drove to Texas to complete preparations there, then turned around and drove to Rochester, where they spent a brief honeymoon on Dr. Will's Mississippi boat, the North Star. Edith told Chuck, "I think you will love Ruth, for she is a sensible and beautiful girl; and I think she will be a great asset in Joe's life. Joe has something to work for that is worth while. Ruth is very domestic and has unusually good taste, and too she has a fine background. Her parents are devoted to each other and to their children and home and are, as well, good citizens and very much respected by everybody."

Two weeks after Joe's wedding, on Saturday, June 25, Chuck married Alice in a large ceremony in Philadelphia. Like Ruth, Alice was 19 when she married. Joe arrived from a happy honeymoon to be best man for his brother. Esther came from Choate School to be Alice's bridesmaid, and little Sally was flower girl.

Chuck and Alice married at four in the afternoon in the Tully Memorial Presbyterian Church, which was "profusely decorated with flowers, palms and ferns," according to the *Rochester Post Bulletin*. Alice wore a "beautiful old fashioned gown of ivory satin and tulle, trimmed with old Brussels lace" and a veil of Dutchess lace. She carried roses, orchids and lilies of the valley. After the ceremony, "a brilliant and festive reception was held at the fashionable Green Hills farm in Overbrook in an exquisite summery setting."

Describing Alice, the newspaper reporter added, "She visited Rochester last spring….Her personality and gentleness of manner gained her a wide circle of friends who will welcome her return." After a short honeymoon, Chuck brought his bride to live in Ivy Cottage, the first dwelling his father had built on the Mayowood property, and Chuck began work in postgraduate surgical training at the Clinic.

Edith still had five children living at home – Dorothy, Louise, Esther, John and Sally. By now she had eased her methods of rearing marriageable girls. She allowed young men to pick up Esther in their cars and take her to town dances. One young man who liked doing this was H. Frederic Helmholz, Jr., who was two years younger than Esther. He described Esther as "a rascal. She had a lovely touch of madness."

Since Esther was never ready for dates on time, Edith waited with Fred. Speaking of this experience 70 years later, Dr. Helmholz remembered Edith's gracious manner of leading the conversation to his life and interests, not her own. She wanted to get to know him.

By the second summer, Fred was becoming more interested in Esther. That was when Edith gave him "the wisdom of age," which he accepted and appreciated.

Edith had discovered that Fred, the son of a doctor, had ambitions to follow his father's path. But in 1927 he was only 16 and Esther 18. He still had high school, college and medical school to go before he could think of marrying.

"Esther's not going to wait for you," Edith counseled. "And if you gave up your future hopes for her, she would know it, and you wouldn't forget it either." It was the same advice Edith was giving her son Joe that springtime——finish your medical training before you marry. But in Helmholz's case, Edith's advice was accepted because of its obvious correctness. When Helmholz did marry, in September, 1935, he chose Dr. Will's granddaughter, Mary Damon Balfour, as his wife. Edith sent a warm note. "I'm glad you're still in the family," she said.

Louise, Edith's next child to marry, chose Tuesday, April 10, 1928, for her wedding to George Treat Trenholm of St. Paul, Minnesota. Always an independent thinker, Louise had said she would never marry a doctor; George worked for a bus company.

Like her sister, Louise wanted her wedding to be in the Big House. Once more, Edith managed the event. According to the local newspaper, the setting was beautiful: silver vase-shaped baskets of pink roses and Easter lilies, placed at intervals in two rows with white satin ribbons looped between them, created an aisle for the bridal party's processional. Louise wore an Empire

style gown of ivory grosgrain silk with a flaring Medici collar. Her veil, created from the wedding veils of her sister Edith and her sister-in-law Alice, was edged with rosepoint lace. It covered her face, falling from a crown decorated with orange blossoms and pearls, and hung in two tiers in back, the longer tier falling to the train of her gown. She carried a bouquet of lilies of the valley, maiden hair ferns and lavendar orchids. A new minister at Calvary Episcopal Church, the Reverend Guy C. Menefee, performed the ceremony.

Attending Louise were her sisters Edith, Esther, and Sally as flower girl. Little Buck, now four, was train-bearer. George chose his brother, Arthur Trenholm, Jr., and Dr. Chuck as his attendants.

After the wedding reception, Louise and George left for a short wedding trip. Then they settled into a home in St. Paul. By now, Edith and Dr. Charlie were looking for a house Joe and Ruth could live in when they returned in early summer from their year in Texas.

Edith was happy. Though her chickens had flown the nest, they hadn't landed far away. Her children and grandchildren remained in easy communication, and in the autumn of 1928, Louise and George came to Rochester to live after George bought a city bus company. In time, they settled in "White Gables," and the Rankins moved to a big house in town.

During the late twenties and early thirties – happy years – Edith set for herself the task of training Dr. Chuck's new wife, Alice, to someday take her place at Mayowood. Being very young, Alice had much to learn before she would be ready to manage the Big House and act as official hostess to a Doctor Mayo after Dr. Charlie retired. Because Chuck followed his father's example and, in his sister Louise's words, "worked like a dog," Alice was alone much of the time. Chuck rose at five each morning, made rounds of his patients, reported to the chief surgeon, assisted in surgery all day, and then made rounds again to check on his postoperative patients. At night, he was on call for emergencies. Edith began including Alice in her own activities, and Alice appreciated her mother-in-law's efforts. In wonder, Alice once told Chuck, "She makes me feel that I'm indispensable!"

Edith's plan was to consult Alice about decisions as if Alice had more knowledge than she. Dr. Chuck wrote, "It was a demonstration of tact typical of my mother, not too common anywhere, but maybe especially rare, I've been told, in mothers-in-law."

By now the Big House was slowly filling up with beautiful and expensive works of art, many of them purchased on Edith and Dr. Charlie's European trips. Although she loved beautiful objects and lived in a luxurious home filled with them, Edith never forgot the simple farm background she came from. Her

granddaughter Mayo described her as being "so homespun….[This was the] main thing about her. She fit in with kings and scrub ladies. Everyone was equal in her eyes. She could speak her mind with the best, but, you know, she never lost the home grown, down-on-the-farm simplicity, calm, and delight in everything….She hated anyone to make a fuss over her."

One day Alice was helping Edith wash, dry, and put away some expensive china. Alice learned about Edith's down-on-the-farm simplicity when, according to Dr. Chuck, "she accidentally broke an irreplaceable procelain cup. She was horrified and on the verge of tears, but Mother comforted her. 'Don't worry, my dear,' she said. 'it is only material.'"

Edith's priority system was operating perfectly. She continued to support the Mayo Clinic however she could and still lavished time on her husband, children, children-in-law, grandchildren, and friends. The family continued growing. By September of 1928, Edith had five grandchildren, all living near the Big House. She managed to see them often.

Dr. Will announced his retirement from surgery on July 1, 1928. His powers were undiminished, but he was developing a slight tremor, and he wanted to retire "while I'm still good," he said. He continued to work every day at the Clinic in a consulting capacity. According to the Clinic business manager, Harry

Harwick, Dr. Will's "great surgical skill was not entirely wasted,…for he often scrubbed and went into operating rooms to lecture as others operated. In fact, some surgeons believe that the Mayos' greatest contributions as teachers came after they had retired from active surgery."

Dr. Will's timing was good, for a crowning achievement was about to occur at the Clinic, one which had taken two years to develop – the new 15-story Plummer Building was opening. (It supplemented the Mayo Building of 1914, which was already much too small.) On September 16, Dr. Will dedicated its 23 bell carillon, which hung in a four-story tower. In all, the bells weighed 36,988 pounds. He dedicated them "to the American soldier, in grateful memory of heroic actions on land and sea to which America owes her liberty, peace, and prosperity."

There was no formal opening ceremony for the structure. The carillon dedication, Dr. Charlie said, had to suffice: "Because of the great necessity of using the new Clinic Building as rapidly as the floors are completed,… the Clinic is declared open." It cost three million dollars, contained examining rooms, research rooms, an X-ray section, and laboratories. A beautiful structure of peach Siena stone and Indiana limestone, it was richly ornamented. Two solid bronze outer doors, weighing 4,000 pounds each and standing 16 feet high, marked the building's entrance. They were originally intended to

close each night, but they have remained open. Only to show special honor are they ever closed, as they were for the funerals of Dr. Henry Plummer, Dr. Charlie, Dr. Will, Dr. Balfour, Dr. Chuck, and President John F. Kennedy.

In the autumn of 1928, Edith and Dr. Charlie sent their daughter Esther to the Florentine School in Florence, Italy, a finishing school for young women. Separations were always difficult for Edith. She wrote Esther faithfully each week, as she had always written each of her children when they were away from her. Edith's habit of prayer helped her endure her daughter's absence:
"Dearest of Esthers,

"…A little prayer for your safety goes out of our window (and I pray it in some way reaches the dear Lord) every night – a prayer that you may be given wisdom and strength to overcome all temptations and always keep your own self respect. I open the curtains and imagine I am looking at you in your little bed – always asleep, because you are six hours ahead of us."

Esther was the last child born to Edith, and she was both beautiful and adventurous. Edith worried about several dangers:

"I want you to keep well, because I cannot bear to think of you ill and away from me. Use good judgment always – think before you act. You say you have gone horseback riding; I hardly blame you, for it is a great pastime and exercise, and I am not going to ask you not to do it again – but take no chances with either horses or men. Safety First.

"Always the same devoted,
"Mother."

The following summer, Dr. Charlie went to Germany, accompanied by his surgical assistant, Dr. John Berry Hartzell, a young Clinic fellow who was fluent in German. From there, the men traveled to Italy, where they met Esther, now finished with her work at the Florentine School and ready to join them in some European travel. The first time Dr. Hartzell saw Esther, in Venice, she was running after pigeons in St. Mark's Square, trying to kick them. (This is a story often retold in the Hartzell family).

Edith joined the group in Italy, and they traveled on to Manchester, England, where they met Dr. Will, Hattie, and the brothers' sister Gertrude. On July 24, the University of Manchester conferred honorary doctor of law degrees on Dr. Charlie and Dr. Will, and the next day the three siblings presented a stained glass window in their father's honor to St. Mary's Church in the Eccles parish, near Manchester. (Dr. W. W. Mayo had been born in Eccles and attended St. Mary's as a boy.) It was a rare occasion, because Dr. Will, Dr. Charlie and Gertrude traveled together.

This was the last long trip Dr. Charlie was able to make in perfect health. On January 2, 1930, he suddenly became dizzy while operating. "His retirement from surgery came abruptly," Dr. Chuck said. For the first time, Dr. Chuck was acting as his father's first assistant; he completed the operation.

When examined at the Clinic, Dr. Charlie was told he had suffered a retinal hemorrhage. He recovered, but he never again performed surgery.

Soon afterwards, Edith phoned Dr. Chuck at night and asked him to come immediately to the Big House. Dr. Charlie had suffered a stroke. It was not severe, and though he was temporarily paralyzed on his right side, he recovered with what Dr. Chuck called "only slight impairment to speech and his extraordinary mental agility." Soon Dr. Charlie was again reporting every day to his office in the new Plummer Building, acting as a surgical consultant and dealing with his vast correspondence.

On September 6, 1930, Esther Mayo married Dr. John Hartzell, attended by a large wedding party, including both her brothers, Dr. Chuck and Dr. Joe. Her flower girl was four-year-old Missey Rankin, and her ring-bearer six-year-old Buck.

Esther's wedding, performed by the Reverend Guy Menefee, took place before 200 guests in Calvary Episcopal Church. According to the *Rochester Post Bulletin*, "Ferns, smilax and palms were massed in the organ and choir lofts, transforming the chancel into a bower of greenery." Esther's gown was of old ivory satin with a V-shaped neckline and long sleeves. A court train fell from soft circular folds in back, and her tulle veil was held by a cap of rosepoint lace. She carried her

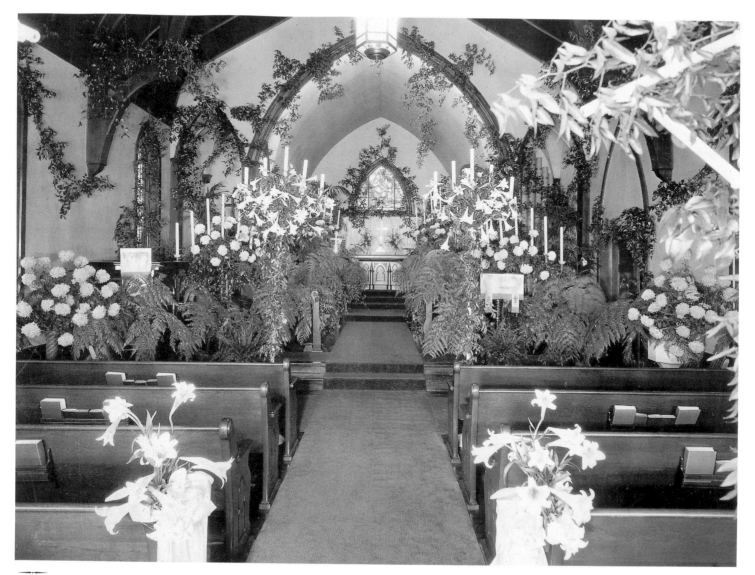

mother's gift, a small, white leather prayerbook, interlaced with tiny gold ribbons to which lilies of the valley were tied. Autumn colors of gold and brown were used in sanctuary flowers and the attendants' dresses.

James Drummond played a concert of organ music during the wedding ceremony. Shortly before the bridal party exited the church, he walked the short block to the Plummer Building, climbed to its carillon tower, and at the proper moment, played the Lohengrin Bridal chorus on the bells as the wedding party recessed. Their music sounded over the town.

Drummond played organ music again in the Big House as the newly married couple greeted their reception guests. Then dinner was served in the courtyard, decorated in the same gold and brown colors as the wedding, including sheaves of farm grains just harvested from the Mayo farms.

When Esther had written her parents in March, asking permission to marry Dr. John, Edith replied for them both,
"My precious girl,…You say you are sure your heart is directing you, and that John is the only man in the world for you (or words to that effect). That is all the assurance we need….If

you find yourself wondering if you are going to be able to make John happy and not wondering if you are going to be happy and contented yourself, it is the right sort of love – the kind that will last through trials and tribulations. Love is sacrifice from beginning to end – sweet sacrifice though….Be happy. To be supremely loved by a good man is the sweetest thing in the world. You both have our blessings.
"Deeply,
"Mother."

Esther and Dr. John honeymooned on a two week motor trip through New England and then moved to their home in Detroit, Michigan, where Dr. John began his private surgical practice with Dr. J. Walter Vaughan, formerly of Rochester. Esther was Edith's only child living away from home.

Life was good and full of adventure for Edith at this time. She wrote Esther one month after the wedding to report on an afternoon's fun: "I had a wonderful fly yesterday with a young aviator (patient) who has the best looking plane I've ever seen. [We went] all over this creation. Enjoyed it a lot."

Early in 1931, she decided to take a "splendid spree" with Dorothy. They left Rochester on January 31, traveling to New York City and Washington, D.C.; from there by ship to Cuba, and then through the Panama Canal to San Francisco, where they were met by the family's chauffeur, who drove them north through California to Portland, Oregon, and then south to Los

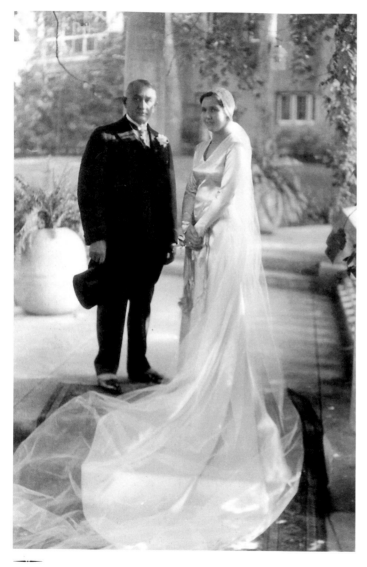

Angeles, where they met Dr. Charlie. With him, they enjoyed a restful, happy trip through Yosemite National Park, returning home to Rochester the end of April. Throughout the 1930's, Edith and Charlie traveled to the Southwest during Minnesota's winter months.

Edith's family was prospering and growing; by early 1931, young Edith had four children, Chuck two, and Louise two. But one married couple remained childless – Dr. Joe and Ruth. Joe was by now in the midst of his fellowship in medicine at the Mayo Clinic. He and Ruth lived in a white house with a red roof across the Zumbro River from the Big House, clearly visible from the living room windows. Because of Ruth's diabetes, she was not expected to be able to have children. According to Dr. Chuck, though, "with her warm nature she was anxious to try, despite the hopelessness of it." She conceived three baby boys; they were all born dead. So Ruth and Joe decided to adopt a baby who had been born December 31, 1930; they named him David.

In the summer of 1932, Edith settled a question Dorothy had been repeatedly asking her for years:

"What is going to happen to me? The other girls are marrying and moving away. When will my turn come?"

Edith's ambitions for Dorothy were that she might live as normal a life as possible. Dorothy understood that her sisters and brothers had moved away and were living with other people. She knew her sisters received diamond rings and were guests of honor at showers before they moved. As usual, Edith did the best she could for Dorothy. She herself bought Dorothy a diamond ring. This was not a small, inconspicuous stone. Dorothy's ring, a European cut diamond of one and three-quarters carats, was set in white gold, with six small diamonds inlaid in a single row down each side of the shank.

Edith gave Dorothy a shower too, inviting many friends and suggesting they give gifts suitable for a young woman's apartment. In a carriage house behind one of the Grahams' houses in Rochester, Edith rented an apartment and furnished it. Then with her parents' love and good wishes, Dorothy moved to her apartment, where she was cared for by a cousin, Frances Graham McClure, daughter of Edith's brother Arthur Graham and his wife Susie. Frances was a widow, only one year younger than Dorothy, with a five-year-old son, Benjamin McClure, Jr., to care for. She was grateful to accept the task of caring for her cousin during the week. On weekends, Dorothy would often go back to the Big House, to be with her mother,

father, and the rest of the family.

Edith's grandchildren, as they grew up, enjoyed entertaining Dorothy. Charles Rankin remembered one day when "I took Dorothy bowling. She had never bowled before. I taught her the basic procedure and then sent two balls down the lane to show her what to do. She picked up her first ball and more or less held it in both hands, and s-l-o-w-l-y took about ten short steps. Then she just dropped the ball on the lane. Her ball headed s-l-o-w-l-y to the right gutter but kept on the lane. At the right moment, the ball headed left and did its job, striking the head pin and the one behind simultaneously. Very s-l-o-w-l-y one by one, all the pins went down. Everyone in the place saw that strike and gave her a rousing cheer."

Dorothy loved sledding and tobogganing with her nieces and nephews. Each Christmas she knitted a scarf, cap, mittens, or socks for each of them. Muff remembered Dorothy, who was always happy it seemed, "interrupting and happily babbling away at solemn family occasions" until someone, often Esther, told her impatiently to be quiet, or Granny, more gently said, "Now, that's enough!"

The autumn and winter of 1932 were difficult for Edith. Dr. Fred Rankin, her son-in-law, planned to leave the Clinic and return to a surgery practice in Lexington, Kentucky. He was a brilliant surgeon who later became president of the American Medical Association. But Dr. Will and the Board of Governors found, in Dr. Chuck's words, "his temperament… unsuited to the cooperative mood of group practice, and he left the Clinic, with the customary severance gift of a year's pay." According to Missey Rankin Redden, "It was undoubtedly better for my father [to leave]. He needed to be on his own and not part of a group."

Edith was pained by this decision. She cherished the companionship of her daughter, son-in-law, and their four children. For a second time, her priority system was shaken and her affections came down on the side of family. Dr. Chuck said, "Mother turned to me and urged me to demonstrate family loyalty by resigning from the Board [of Governors]. I, however, had learned Father's strategy in such emergencies, and I kept quiet and waited out the storm. The Rankins left town and Uncle Will…was designated a villain, a role he bore with equanimity until Mother got over her indignation."

Covering her anger and sorrow, Edith invited 30 of Dr. Rankin's friends to the Big House on Saturday, December 17, 1932, to an elegant goodbye party for the departing couple. She chose a "Gay Nineties" theme and furnished some costumes from her own fancy dresses of 40 years earlier, when she was a newly married woman. Edith herself wore a formal ivory satin gown, with an ivory lace skirt draped over the satin underskirt and a matching lace scarf about her shoulders. Young Edith wore a fancy dress from the '90's of white dotted tulle with dropped shoulders, a lace collar, and black velvet bows trimming the skirt. One of Edith's 40-year-old dresses of black taffeta with puffed sleeves and ruffles at the hem looked dramatic on Ruth. Even the men got into the spirit of the nineties, wearing Prince Albert coats with ascot ties and brightly colored vests. James Drummond came to the party dressed as Little Lord Fauntleroy.

Edith hired an orchestra to provide dance music in the ballroom, and late in the evening, she presided at the buffet supper. *The Rochester Post Bulletin* reported, "The revival of trousseaux and wardrobes of other days…contrived to make the ball a brilliant social affair." In this way, Edith and Dr. Charlie parted with their daughter, Dr. Fred, and their four grandchildren, who left in early January, 1933, for Kentucky.

About this time, Dr. Charlie, who had been musing on the problem of diabetic women losing their babies, counseled Ruth and Joe to try again. He figured Ruth could bear a live baby if delivered early by Caesarian section. "Ruth gamely agreed," according to Dr. Chuck. She went into the hospital for observation during her fourth month of pregnancy and stayed there in bed until the seventh month, when she was successfully delivered of a healthy baby boy on August 16, 1933. (This method of helping diabetic women bear live babies was widely imitated afterwards.) Ruth and Joe named their son William James Mayo II, after Dr. Will.

Also in 1933 Robin Trenholm was born, the fourth child of Louise and George Trenholm. He was a "blue baby" and died hours after birth. Edith was traveling when she heard the news and wrote a letter of consolation to her grieving daughter, assuring her the baby had gone straight to heaven. She said, "You, Louise, have a wonderful family of children and your art, and you will move on, just as I did many years ago. Today is for the living, and you have so much to give the world."

⁓

When Edith was lonely for those who were away, she would find new people to befriend. She was always looking for someone to help and encourage. One miserable snowy day a little boy named Neil Mahoney was walking home from the Bamber Valley School. Suddenly a big car, driven by a chauffeur, stopped on the road, and Edith leaned out the window to ask Neil if he'd like a ride. He climbed right in. She was shocked to see his bare hands, head and neck – he was covered only by his coat. After he'd warmed up in the car, she dropped him off at his house. The next day the Mahoney family received – anonymously – a big box of new wool mittens, scarves, socks and knit caps for their seven children. They were grateful always but puzzled about who gave the gift. Many years later

Edith's granddaughter Mayo received a beautiful letter from Neil, now grown to manhood, saying he had finally figured out the "connection between Granny and that cold day….He added that his respect for her was immense."

⁓

On Wednesday, August 8, 1934, the weather in Rochester was not what a hostess would choose for the most important dinner party of her life. Edith was planning to entertain President Franklin Delano Roosevelt. The day dawned hot and sultry. Showers fell in Wabasha County, and "a furious storm" lashed Winona on the banks of the Mississippi to the east, according to the *Rochester Post Bulletin*. Then clouds over Rochester broke to let the sun shine through. By mid-afternoon the temperature climbed to 97 humid degrees. It was a day to melt gelatin salads and floating custard desserts before they could be brought to the table.

Dr. Charlie had long ago designed the Big House with insulating air spaces between its poured concrete walls and a fan system to blow cooler air from the hill cabins into the house. These helped somewhat. Edith managed to adjust her dinner menu so the food could be served with some elegance even in the terrible heat.

For weeks, many people had been working to make Mayowood ready. Outside, straggly annual plants were uprooted and replaced with luxuriantly flowering geraniums, and the lawn was trimmed to perfection. Inside, all the carpets were removed and rubber mats installed beneath them, to accommodate the President's moving about: both his legs were braced with metal, a necessity because they were paralyzed from polio.

At 10 in the morning the President's train arrived in town. He was welcomed by a giant throng as his car drove down Broadway, a crowd which stretched over 67 blocks and was estimated at 75,000 people. Approximately 8,000 people, including "many of the country's medical and civilian great," according to Clapesattle, gathered under the scorching sun in Soldiers Field. F.D.R. had come to present an award from the American Legion, honoring Dr. Charlie and Dr. Will for the free medical and surgical treatment of World War I veterans they had offered at the Clinic since the war. He gave them a plaque and spoke, both to the assembled crowd and to a nationwide audience over radio. The Minnesota American Legion commander, M. F. Murray, also thanked Dr. Will and Dr. Charlie. For many people, Clapesattle said, this day "honoring the beloved brothers seemed…the culminating triumph of their career."

The American Legion award was more personal to Dr. Charlie and Edith than people knew. Their daughter Louise had been asked to sculpt two medallions, one of her father and one of her Uncle Will, which she barely managed to complete in time.

She made them in clay, then drove to Minneapolis to the foundry, where they were bronzed and set into the larger bronze memorial of the occasion.

After the ceremony, Dr. Will, Dr. Charlie and President Roosevelt were driven in an open car to the Big House. To the dismay of the President's guards, Dr. Charlie changed the route at the last minute, instructing the chauffeur to drive out into the country so the President could see the new medical research center the Clinic was building.

At Mayowood, Edith welcomed the President and other guests. She entered the large dining room on the President's arm, leading the procession of well-dressed diners. Along with the President at the head table were seated Dr. Charlie and Edith, Dr. Will and Hattie, Edith's brother Dr. Kit and Blanche, Edith's sister Dinah Olin and Dr. Charlie's sister Gertrude Berkman, (both women now widows), and seven other distinguished people, members of the President's party and the president of the railroad on which the President traveled. At a second table were seated the President's son John Roosevelt and Edith and Charlie's children and their Mayo cousins plus members of the Presidential party.

Dr. Charlie was immensely pleased with the events. The next day he spoke publicly, "The President has come and gone. Our great day is over, but its memory will always remain; it all adds to our affection for our comrades, the members of the American Legion, who worked so hard to make the event possible. To say much would be an anticlimax, but it was the greatest public event in my life, and I appreciated what was done for me."

The famous American humorist Will Rogers was a friend of Dr. Charlie. People said the two men could have been brothers, their speaking style – slow and humorous – might have been learned from the same parents. One evening, Dr. Charlie and Edith read in the paper that Will Rogers was sick. That night Dr. Charlie woke suddenly and said to Edith, "Will wants me."

"Now, why would he want you now?" she asked, thinking he meant his brother.

"No. Will Rogers wants me," he said, and shortly after, a call came from Rogers, asking for medical advice.

This was not unusual for Dr. Charlie. He was sometimes prescient about patients, waking in the night, dressing, and hurrying to the hospital to discover that his intuition was correct: the person he was concerned about had taken a turn for the worse, and Dr. Charlie arrived just in time to help or to simply, quietly, hold the patient's hand. According to Louise Mayo Trenholm, "He couldn't bear it when someone died and was all alone."

In the thirties, Edith entertained famous people in addition to F.D.R. and Will Rogers. The King of Nepal stayed at the Big House. Helen Keller became a personal friend. One day Keller and her companion were with Edith in her living room, over by the windows. All three white-haired ladies, according to Mayo, were "leaning forward with hands touching lips and fingers working furiously in hands. All of a sudden something funny was said, and all three started to laugh. Their heads were all bent in towards each other, almost touching. Each put a hand to her mouth, as if to laugh out loud quietly and politely behind their hands, and all three bounced up and down with their giggles....I [the child observing] did not know that Helen Keller could not hear or see. At that moment all were equal and understood the joke."

Edith's relationship with her grandchildren was close. She treasured each of them. As the years went by, a tradition developed between Granny and the Trenholm children. Mayo described it: "Every Mother's Day Granny would come down early for breakfast at White Gables. It was a big deal....Great preparation went on during the previous days. We children would go up among the black walnut trees above the farm and pick the new gorgeous violets, one of her favorite flowers. It seemed to take a long time, hours and hours, until our little pails were full. We would lay the violets out in cups of water, and we braided them one by one,...until we had a very long rope. This would be worked together into a four inch band with a big hole in the center——the entire crown. We would scream with delight....

"After baths, clean clothes, tightly braided hair, and smiles, we would carry this – wet, cold (it would have been in the icebox for two days), in to Granny. She would be sitting in a special chair, in a special place. She would be sitting with her hands folded, waiting for what I am sure was a terrible ordeal. We would sing, and she would wait. We would dance, and she would wait, with that little smile on her face. George [the eldest Trenholm child] would carry the wreath on a gorgeous white lace pillow and carefully bow in front of her. I would take the wreath and lift it up on her head. By now the pillow was wet. The wreath, drooping a bit, would seem heavy and almost too much for me. What if I dropped it?

"And there she would sit, that smile on her face, and become the very special mother of all time. All morning she would sit with that terribly heavy, ugly mess of flowers. The water would drip down her face, the loose flowers hang down onto her neck. She never complained and in the end told each of us how special we were and how precious she felt."

Chapter 8

THE FINAL YEARS

Will Rogers – only 56 – was killed in a plane crash near Point Barrow, Alaska, on August 15, 1935, beginning what became, for Edith, a series of terrible deaths.

This sad event was followed the same year by another unexpected, sudden death. Dr. E. Starr Judd died on November 30 of virulent pneumonia, while on a trip to Chicago to see a football game. He was 57, head of the surgical staff at the Clinic, and one of the original partners. In 1903 he had been first assistant to Dr. Charlie; in 1904 he was appointed head of his own surgical section – the first surgeon besides the Mayo brothers to have such authority. His parting was unexpected and deeply felt. Not only was he important to the Clinic, he was also important as a member of the family, since he was Dr. Charlie's nephew by marriage. His wife Helen was the daughter of Gertrude Mayo Berkman.

But for Edith, the most grievous death occurred on November 9, 1936. Her son Dr. Joe was found dead near Alma, Wisconsin, after what appeared to be a terrible car-train accident. He had been duck-hunting on the last day of the season and afterwards had eaten dinner in a small hotel, then gambled, playing poker with some other men. Then he apparently drove off towards home with his golden retriever, Foosie, beside him in the car. The first issue of a new magazine, *Life*, reported: "To make a short cut from one highway to another, Dr…Mayo…drove along the Burlington Railroad tracks….Before Dr. Mayo had bumped a mile over the ties, an express train came roaring along at 65 m.p.h." and hit his car, which was carried "half a mile back along the right of way." This train, from Chicago, approached from behind; in the darkness, the engineer didn't see the car until it was too late; the car was cut in two. Both Dr. Joe and Foosie were found dead. People theorized that thickly falling snow that night obscured Joe's vision, causing him to mistake the railroad track for a road.

The family withheld one fact from the reporters. Foosie didn't die from a car/train wreck: a bullet was found in her head. Dr. Chuck traveled several times to Wisconsin to investigate the accident and learned that Joe had won a great deal of money that night. However, no money was found on his body. Some of the family always suspected Joe was murdered, with robbery the motive. Since the men Joe had gambled with were long gone from the scene, these suspicions were impossible to prove. Edith's granddaughter Mayo pointed to another factor that influenced them: "How strong this family was. They didn't push an investigation for fear it would affect the Clinic." Once more Edith's priority system had been tested, and she kept the Clinic a top priority.

Joe had said for months before his death, almost like

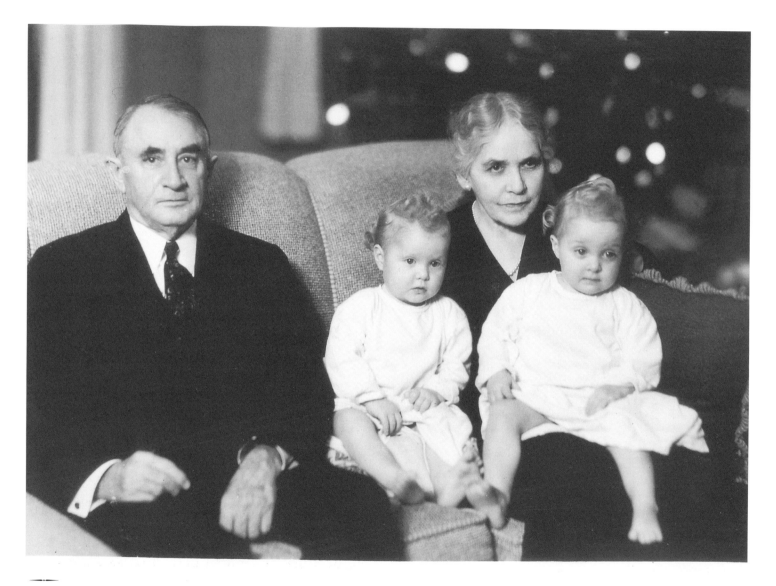

a prediction, "When I die, I want to be buried with my dog." This request Dr. Charlie, Edith, Ruth, and Dr. Chuck decided to honor, especially since Joe and Foosie had been nearly inseparable in life. The minister who conducted the funeral service at Mayowood objected to performing it over a casket which held a dog. Finally, he was persuaded to do it.

Mayo described the service from her six-year-old perspective: "I stared at [Uncle Joe] in his coffin. My eyes were level with him, and the dog's face came up over his shoulder. It was a very large coffin, and they had taken leaves and scattered them all over him. He looked as if he were a Snow White counterpart before the prince came with a kiss.

"Granny came over and we stood there for a long time, with her arm over my shoulder. I asked her if we could kiss him and wake him up. 'No,' she said. I asked if we could shake him. Would he wake up? 'No,' she said. I told her he was my favorite uncle and I would miss him. She said he was one of her favorite sons and she would miss him too."

This son Edith once described with the words,

"Joseph, dear, you have a few faults, and we will work on them, but you have the most amazing gift – your love for people and their uncanny delight in you. This is a gift no one can give you, and you wear it as easily as your clothes."

Joe was the only one of Edith's children with the nerve to treat Dr. Will playfully. Esther told a story about Dr. Will riding in the front of a crowded elevator, with Dr. Joe several people deep behind him. Spontaneously, Joe reached forward and pinched Dr. Will on his behind, then faked innocence when the stern, authoritative Will turned around in amazement.

Dr. Chuck said about losing his brother "half of me died with him….When he died, I lost the only person who really knew what I am and what I faced. I was left alone with the whole weight of being a Mayo successor. Until then, it had been easier to keep up my courage because Joe's irreverence cut through my gloomy self-consciousness and made me chuckle."

In keeping with what Edith had taught him about courtesy to the suffering, Dr. Chuck mastered his grief enough to write, eleven days after his brother's death, a letter to the engineer in charge of the train which had struck Joe's car. It was written "from the deepest place in my heart….For myself and for the family, I express to you our most sincere good wishes and the hope that you will carry on in the responsible position which you occupy and not let an accident in which you had an

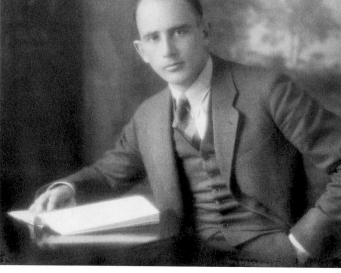

An image of Joe made shortly before his death

Photo courtesy of Mayo Kooiman

woods, riding their horses, and the pack of hunting dogs running ahead and behind, all yapping. I can hear her throaty laugh – drifting right out into the air as if it were meant just for me to hear, so I might remember it. It was very infectious, and oh, was she gorgeous."

When Joe died, he was 34, Ruth only 28. Their two little boys were five (David) and three (Billy).

Eight weeks after Joe's death, on December 31, 1936, Dr. Henry Plummer became ill early in the afternoon. He diagnosed himself with cerebral thrombosis, a blood clot in the brain. Plummer asked his driver to take him to the Plummer Building. Somehow, he managed to slowly walk around the first floor. He calmly examined the bronze doors, the rich marble floors and walls. He sat in the long hall for a long time and gazed at the beauty of the building he had designed. Then he was driven home. He called for his family to come immediately and predicted he would lose consciousness within the hour, which he did. He died the next night, age 62. Again, as with Dr. Judd, his loss was felt both at the Clinic and in the family. His wife was Daisy Berkman, Dr. Charlie's niece.

innocent part affect you too much."

Edith's grief remained intense for a long time, but she had learned, with the deaths of little Margaret, Rachel and many others by this time, the discipline of looking forward, not backward, and of focusing her attention on the living. The one who needed help most was Joe's widow, Ruth. According to Mayo, "Ruth was devastated when Joe died. Ruth and Joe were madly in love. Both were heavy on the emotions….They loved their drinks, dogs, horses, and hunting. I can still hear them laughing in the

Dr. Plummer's influence on the Mayo Clinic was profound; he designed the medical records system – a significant contribution to the Clinic's superior health care – and he also gave his architecture and engineering knowledge to the design of both the 1914 Mayo Building and the 1928 Plummer Building. Besides this, he was an extraordinary doctor, making discoveries which contributed to medical knowledge, according to Clark Nelson, in "hematology, roentgenology, bronchoscopy, esophagoscopy, electrocardiography, and to knowledge of the physiology and pathology of the thyroid gland." Dr. Will always said Dr. Plummer was of first importance to the development of the Clinic after Dr. Charlie and himself.

To escape the rigorous Minnesota winter and to try to recover from these losses, Dr. Charlie and Edith traveled with Dr. Will and Hattie to the American Southwest in early 1937. They had gone the previous winter too, on a trip which included Dr. Kit and Blanche. On Edith's seventieth birthday, February 12, 1937, Kit wrote her from Rochester, remembering the year before: "I see you motoring here and there, from city to city, to mountains, up canyons, through deserts! I hope you have soft breezes and mild sunshine to accompany the trips and make the days as glorious as were the days of 1936 when we swept the joyous west with you and had the greatest vacation of our lives!"

He added to the birthday letter an expression of love for his sister, "You are, and have been, one of the great joys and comforts of my life."

Ruth Mayo never recovered completely from the loss of Dr. Joe. Edith tried to comfort her, and so did Louise, who spent many hours with Ruth at this time, mostly on Louise's boat, the "Laisy Daisy." There she engaged Ruth in talking and singing, to divert Ruth's thoughts. When the two women weren't on the Laisy Daisy, they spent time on Ruth's boat, the "Blue Wren."

Edith had always believed in prayer as a source of comfort and strength, and, during these years, she turned to it often. Mayo noted, "You know she was extremely religious. She prayed every night. Her little stand up prayer kneeler was recovered many times. I can see her back, bent over the arm cushion of her kneeler, as she concentrated and whispered quietly."

She also had another place of refuge – the log house built years earlier, which was down along the lake, only a ten minute walk from the Big House. A dwelling of a single room with a bed, table, fireplace, and corner cupboard holding a few dishes, it was built near a spring of clear, fresh water which could be used to cool foods, if Edith planned a long stay. When she needed to be alone, she would retreat to this place, which she called her "crying house."

Muff Mayo remembered asking her mother,

"Where's Granny?"

"She's gone to the log cabin. Don't go looking for her there."

Another source of comfort to Edith was her dedication to the Clinic and her knowledge that it was thriving, and that the people there were doing a sacred task. Once, Edith had written her daughter Esther advice from her own life experience, "I am sure that you are developing into a wonderful woman – you don't have to be like me or like anybody but yourself....you have great possibilities....I want you to find something that you love to devote yourself to."

This was essentially what Edith, herself, had done. She had found something she loved, and she had devoted herself to it – the work of healing the sick. As the Clinic grew, and as medical knowledge expanded because of Clinic research, Edith took great comfort that her life's tasks were being achieved, even when misfortune struck those she loved.

The research on Vitamin C at Mayo Clinic by Dr. Albert Szent-Gyorgyi von Nagyrapolt resulted in his receiving a Nobel Prize in 1937, which gratified Edith, as did the on-going work of Mayo in establishing the nation's first blood bank for collecting, storing and transfusing blood.

Even with these sources of comfort, however, in November, 1937, Edith grieved afresh over the loss of her son. Characteristically for her, she reached out lovingly to Ruth. In a letter written November 5, Edith said:

"My dear sweet Ruth,

"...Today, the fifth of November, a year ago at noon in Kahler Club, you and Joe with others had lunch with us – the last time I saw my precious son alive. I feel I want to talk with you, his dearest possession. I want to say again that it is sweet to remember and be thankful for all the happy happy times he had. You quite satisfied his soul, I think. David and Biljim [William] added the final touch that made his life quite perfect. He did his job well and would have made a name for himself in medicine and in his own way....I have only sweet and precious memories of Joe through all his life, and I am thankful that he had so much joy and gave so much joy. It can never be quite the same again without him, but I have no bitterness in my heart, only thankfulness that we had him 34 precious years and have you and the boys through him, to love and be loved by. If I didn't love you for yourself, which I do, I'd love you for all you have meant to him, dear Ruth. You have been through a hard year and I do hope that time has helped you, and that you will be able to carry on sturdily for the boys now, and perhaps sometime you will meet someone with whom you could live happily and who would help carry your burdens and make life a little less lonely....

"Again, dear love to you,
"Mother."

The letter reached Ruth at a town along the Mississippi River. She was traveling with friends down

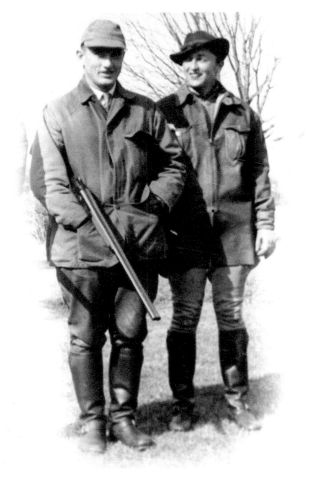

river to New Orleans as chief pilot of the Blue Wren, a rare skill for a woman in her twenties. They left Wabasha, Minnesota, on October 18 and arrived safely in New Orleans November 12. Edith wrote Ruth of the

trip, "It will give you confidence in yourself. It is something to be proud of. I don't know of another girl who could do it."

As more time passed after Joe's death, Dr. Charlie and Edith found relief from sadness in the abundant life they had been creating all along at Mayowood. They both delighted in animals and birds. Dr. Charlie had imported Chinese pheasants and prairie chickens, which were multiplying. He also had been feeding wild geese for some years and, according to Louise, one day "he got cagey." He decided to lure the geese into longer stays. Taking some of his tame female geese, he placed them at the clearing in the woods where wild geese liked to stop, and he loaded this spot with feed grain. It worked well. By 1940, the geese had interbred and multiplied into a flock of about 4,000 geese, who wintered at Mayowood and at Silver Lake near Rochester. Descendants of these geese still live by the thousand in the Rochester area.

Sometimes elk would jump the fence which was supposed to keep them away from the house, but free in the woods. Muff remembered staying overnight at the Big House. "I'd wake up early in the morning and look down on the patio to see sometimes five or six elk near it, browsing on ferns. Then, if something scared them, they would leap the brick wall enclosing it on one side and be off."

In the Big House lived a chihuahua, Peggy, the gift of one of Edith's houseguests. She was an excitable little dog, and when the grandchildren came to visit, Granny would caution, "Children! Children! Speak softly and calmly! You are exciting Peggy!" The dog would streak through the huge living room, dining room and sunroom at top speed and would usually end up vomiting on the rug.

All the other dogs, including a mastiff, lived outdoors. Writing to Esther once, Edith described the mastiff: "I like that four-footed beast, but he is the bane of my life just the same – an ever present pest. He also is treated as one of the family. Your Dad adores him and only grins at all his antics and odors."

There was an indoor parrot, Tony, and an outdoor parrot, Mike, whose swearing was so bad he was shut out in the courtyard in summer and the greenhouse in winter. Muff remembered Tony well, a double yellow head Mexican parrot who lived in his cage in the dining room. When the telephone rang, he would call out, "Mayowood!" right along with the person answering the phone. Edith was careful about her grandchildren's safety around both these birds. She constantly told the youngsters, "Keep your fingers out of their cages or they'll be nipped right off!"

Wild birds continued to delight Edith too. She wrote to Esther telling how thrilled she was with the beauty of birds and flowers. It was March, "very cold but lovely. The other morning the cardinal was outside looking his most beautiful and whistling for all he was worth. It gave me a great thrill to see and hear him, like I get when I find a fringed gentian or hear something in music that seems to come just to me."

To Ruth, Edith wrote, "I could wish for more time to enjoy this beautiful world, which grows more beautiful and more wonderful as we grow older, I think. That is one of the compensations of getting older, and there are very many, believe it or not."

On one occasion, bats got into the Big House and were flying around the living room while little Johnny Hartzell was visiting. "Don't worry about it," Dr. Charlie told him, "they're part of the family."

Dr. Charlie wanted to make a chimpanzee part of the family too, but Edith absolutely refused. This was a creature named Bertha who lived in a tower on the Plummer Building, where she was being used in experimental work which eventually contributed to the discovery of polio vaccine. According to Dr. Chuck, "Bertha adored my father and would embrace him enthusiastically when she saw him, and Father felt affection for her." However, the chimp didn't like Edith. Once, when Edith came to visit her with Dr. Charlie, Bertha seized Edith's purse and tossed it over a parapet, off the tower, where it was difficult to recover.

Bertha might be happier living at Mayowood, Dr.

Charlie suggested, and he even described to Edith how he could easily redo a downstairs bathroom off his study for a comfortable chimp home. Edith vetoed the idea. "If the chimpanzee comes, I go!" she declared.

Edith continued doing kind deeds for suffering neighbors. One day she took her young assistant cook, Brunhilde Brunholzl, with her to visit an elderly couple and their daughter. As the daughter escorted them out afterwards, she confided to Edith, "If I hear one more moan, I don't think I'll be able to take it."

From then on, Edith relieved the daughter regularly, traveling to the house at night, and staying awake to care for the old people so their daughter could sleep. All the staff at the Big House were strictly ordered not to mention this kindness to anyone during Edith's lifetime.

Dr. Chuck remembered, much later, seeing an old man asleep in the sun on the Big House terrace. Edith had taken him in to live with the family, and she personally tended to him until he died, because he had nowhere else to go.

During the late thirties, Edith kept on enjoying her grandchildren. She had a large mahogany dresser with five big drawers in her bedroom; the bottom drawer was exclusively for items the children brought her. Mayo said, "Everyone would leave treasures and gifts to her....What an unbelieveable place it was. You cannot

imagine the precious things to be found – rotten apples, a brown goose egg, terribly dried leaves, snake skins, little rocks, large rocks,...walnuts, flowers long dead and some still only wilted, old dried tomatoes, a small hard pumpkin, a dead mouse, a few dead bugs,...little bits of wood,...some hand-written notes, sometimes a good grade from a school test, a card with 'worked hard' written over from one of the younger children. Everything was important, and the secret is that she did not wish to have the children feel there was not room in her heart for each of them....I can remember walking up [to the Big House] looking everywhere for something special for her. I'm sure the others did too."

Edith would play gin rummy with her grandchildren for hours. By now her hands were so painfully swollen with arthritis, she had difficulty picking up the cards. According to Mayo, "her hands hurt her so much she had to slide the cards from the pile across the table, catch one with the other hand, and lay it on the couch beside her. She couldn't hold the cards." But she had fun playing anyway. She liked to mumble as she played. "Oh! Good for me!" or "Hooray!" would escape her lips, and if her opponent won, it was "Good for Mayo!" or "Good for George!" and "Hooray!" for them.

For the grandchildren, visiting Granny at the Big House was a tremendous treat. Muff was living in Ivy Cottage with her three brothers and sister. Being the oldest of Dr. Chuck's children, she was the one with courage enough to try for overnight stays. She would pack her pajamas in a little suitcase and sneak off up the path to the Big House, where the doors were never locked. She would slip through a door and try to creep up the stairs towards Granny's bedroom, avoiding Anna the housekeeper. If Anna saw Muff, she would always ruin the plan and send her home.

Muff described the adventure: "Stop! Listen! Duck behind a sofa!....It would be glorious when I'd finally hit gold. Granny! I'd immediately ask to spend the night, as I'd always have my suitcase, and she would always say yes. Of course, that included dinner in the big dining room with the innumerable guests."

Edith and Dr. Charlie both appreciated music. When Dr. Charlie interviewed someone to work on his farms, he asked whether the man played a musical instrument, and if so, Dr. Charlie was encouraged to hire him. On summer Sunday afternoons, the family would sit outside on the front terrace to see a small band of farmers come striding up the hill, playing their instruments, led by a trumpeter, the man in charge of chickens. The band would stop below the steps and play a short concert for the family, who would listen and clap, and then Edith would provide food for everyone.

Indoors, much of the music-making happened at the organ in the music room, which could be played as is or turned into an automatic instrument, using preset rolls. Dr. Charlie liked to play the rolls, often with a grandchild sitting with him to help. On Sunday afternoons, James Drummond came out to Mayowood and played the organ by hand. Family and friends came for tea, everyone dressed up. They liked to sing along to the music. Muff remembered "I Was Seeing Nelly Home" as a favorite song.

At Christmastime, a big group of Mayo Clinic fellows always came to the Big House to sing Christmas carols, and Edith would invite the nuns from St. Mary's Hospital to come out and listen with the family.

Christmas day, Drummond played the organ for the big dinner party. He would arrive at the Big House about 4 p.m. to play Christmas music while family and friends – between 100 and 150 people – arrived for drinks preceding dinner. Mayo said the Big House was never overdecorated, but yet, everything was different at Christmastime. It "was truly decorated, but in a different sense. It was colored by the cold outside and the warmth within. It was colored by...all the friendly faces, good cheer, and their red and green finery, the color of huge logs in the fireplace, bowls of nuts to crack and large chunks of fudge on silver plates scattered around on the tables. It was colored by the beautiful silver candelabra, all lit and flickering. Mostly it was colored by all the hugs and kisses, the smiles....The greatest color was watching Granny and Granddaddy walking around and saying something special to everyone."

At a certain time, Drummond would stop playing Christmas music and disappear. Soon sleigh bells would be heard, and Santa Claus would stomp heavily up the entrance steps, laughing. All the children ran to the music room to speak with Santa, and then he would be gone, and Edith would announce, "Now it is time to eat!" The whole party entered the dining room, decorated by a huge Christmas tree on the west end, covered with sparkling lights. Another giant tree stood in the sunroom – the children's tree, thickly sprinkled with gingerbread cookies and apples. By the end of the holiday, the cookies and apples would be eaten off this tree as far up as small arms could reach.

Other than the dining room tree, and centerpieces for the tables, the main decorating element was food, happy-looking food. On one sideboard would be two huge stuffed turkeys, ready to carve, and dishes of dry dressing. On another was a whole fish garnished with lemon. And on the big table, a roasted whole suckling pig lay on a huge platter with an apple in its mouth. Side dishes were presented in silver serving bowls – potatoes, vegetables, hot rolls and salads.

The living room was little decorated except for the mantle, which held small antique statues of Joseph, Mary, the baby Jesus, and an angel standing on a cloud.

A creche scene stood on a small table – the holy family in a stable, felt-covered cows, donkeys, camels and wise men standing by. This shelter was lighted with a little light bulb, which seemed magical to Muff. "We [children] loved it," she said.

Exiting the Big House on Christmas evening, everyone passed a huge stocking hung on the music room door. It was filled with presents for at least 30 little children; as a child left the house, he or she would take one.

Dr. Charlie and Edith liked gathering the family about them. Every summer the out-of-town grandchildren were invited for extended visits. These were splendid six-week long vacations. Tom Hartzell remembered the fun of rodeos on the racetrack behind the stone barns with his Mayo and Trenholm cousins. He rode in an antique stagecoach from Dr. Charlie's collection of vehicles, pulled by horses, while his Mayo cousins chased alongside on their own horses, dressed as Indians. As they attacked his coach, Tom defended it with a cap pistol, cheered on by Edith and the children's parents, watching from a grandstand.

Edith and Dr. Charlie marked the end of autumn every year with a huge bonfire down by the boathouse. To build the bonfire, grandchildren worked for weeks beforehand, gathering sticks and scrub from the woods. On Halloween night, the family gathered around the fire to roast hot dogs, drink hot chocolate, and sing.

Having fun was a tonic for health as important as medicine, Dr. Charlie believed. Therefore he, along with the Mayo Properties Association, contributed money – about $350,000 altogether – to the town of Rochester in 1938 to build a Civic Auditorium, including an ice-skating rink. Dr. Kit wrote Edith, who was in Tucson, Arizona, to thank her as well as Dr. Charlie when he read in the newspaper of "Charlie's magnificent gift." He said, "Husbands do not and cannot rightly give unless the wives are earnest supporters! We, of our house, want to thank you…quite as warmly as we do Charlie."

Edith's biggest delight, as long as he lived, continued to be Dr. Charlie. Mayo wrote a beautiful vignette of their relationship when Charlie was old and had already suffered several strokes. "I love this small moment," Mayo said. "One day I walked into the dark fire-lit living room up at the Big House. There wasn't a sound, no parrot screaming, no people talking, no radio mumblings….Granddaddy was sitting straight up in a high back rose-colored chair with his little Mexican dog asleep on his lap. His glasses had slipped low on his nose, and his mouth allowed soft air to escape. Granny was leaning over him, with a hand on each arm of the chair. She was staring at him. Her face was about a foot away from his face, and she would tip her head this way and a little that way, then back up a bit and lean

forward again. She raised her head to look at me and then put her fingers to her lips.

"Quickly she walked over to me, put her arm around me, and then turned to look back at Granddaddy. 'Isn't he beautiful?' she said. 'Isn't he the most handsome man?'

"I asked her what she was doing. She said she was memorizing his face 'in case he leaves me first. I want to remember what he looks like.'

"She went on to say how much fun it had been living with this man, how soft and tender he was, and how comfortable she felt standing and staring at him. She said looking at him reminded her of when she first saw him. He had winked at her. She felt he had always been a warm coat, and whatever they did or how far apart they were, she was terribly aware of him and felt that same warmth.

"She took my hand and we walked back over to where he slept. She put her hands back on the chair arms and leaned down towards his face. We stood there in silence, and the funniest thing happened. Granddaddy opened his eyes and smiled and winked. We giggled and hugged him. The dog, Peggy, never stirred on his lap.

"I bring this up because it is not a big thing, only

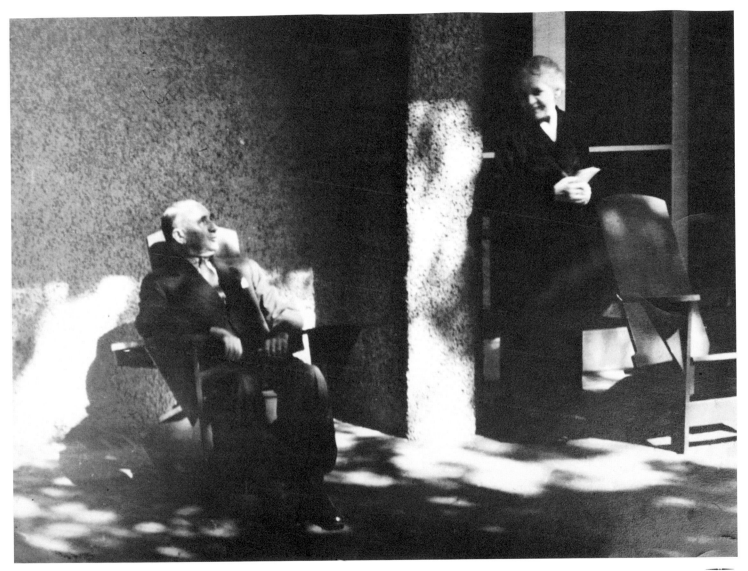

remembering something so small that shows that deep and everlasting attachment they had. I did not know about love, but she was showing me hers."

Dr. Charlie's older sister, Gertrude Mayo Berkman, whom the family called "Auntie Trude," was a source of love and comfort to them over the years. When she died at the age of 85 on July 22, 1938, another series of painful deaths began for Edith.

In 1939 the Mayo Clinic was flourishing. It served its millionth patient. One hundred eighty-seven doctors now made up its medical staff. Only 46 years earlier, when Edith married Dr. Charlie in 1893, its staff totalled three doctors, Dr. Will, Dr. Charlie, and Dr. W. W. Mayo.

The winter months of 1939, Edith and Dr. Charlie spent in Tucson, Arizona, with Dr. Will and Hattie, where each couple owned a western style adobe house with a tile roof. Exactly at eight a.m. each morning, Dr. Will would arrive at Dr. Charlie's house for a visit. At this time Dr. Charlie had trouble walking, because of damage from earlier strokes, but he still had zest for traveling. Edith received a letter which her brother Dr. Kit wrote from Rochester on March 15: "It won't be long until you are all here, perhaps preparing for an English trip!"

In addition to Edith and Dr. Charlie, some of the household staff had traveled to Arizona too, among them Anton Brunholzl, called "Mr. Tony," a skilled carpenter from Germany whose work Dr. Charlie especially admired. Already, in 1939, anti-German sentiment was rising in the United States as people observed Hitler's rise to power. Because of this, Edith made a kind suggestion to Mr. Tony's wife Brunhilde. "I'm called 'Mrs. Charlie,'" Edith said, "and I'm very proud of that. I'm going to call you 'Mrs. Tony,' and you will be very proud of that too." This became the name by which Mrs. Brunholzl was known in the family, from that moment on through all the years she worked in Dr. Charlie's and Dr. Chuck's households.

The Arizona vacation was marred by news that Sister Joseph, superintendent of St. Mary's Hospital and Dr. Will's first assistant for many years, had died on March 29. It was also marred by Dr. Will's ill health. He suffered indigestion, and, believing he might have eaten contaminated food, he and Hattie returned to Rochester early.

Before leaving for Arizona, Edith had spoken to Alice and Chuck, suggesting they go ahead with any ideas they might have to remodel the Big House: "After all," Edith had explained, "you will be living here someday, and you have a right to fix it to suit yourselves."

When Edith returned home, she discovered that Alice and Chuck had, indeed, taken her advice to renovate the Big House. Alice had invented a way to create a cozy and beautiful space for her family, believing that the existing rooms were too large and dark. She had ordered workmen to destroy Edith's study and adjoining bathroom, knocking out walls to create a new room which included the conservatory at the sunny end of the house. In this room workmen placed Minnesota white pine paneling made from doors which Dr. Charlie had purchased when his old elementary school, Rochester Central, was torn down. Alice also designed a windowed alcove and a fireplace, making a beautiful room.

Still, "she was understandably nervous," Dr. Chuck said, on the day Edith and Dr. Charlie returned from Tucson.

Edith had always been a loving mother-in-law to Alice, (as to Ruth), and – put to the test – she passed with a high grade. Dr. Chuck reported, "My mother said at once, and believably, 'I like it, I like it! Alice, how clever you are.'"

However, bad news was on hand in Rochester. Dr. Will was diagnosed at the Clinic with stomach cancer, ironically, his surgical specialty. On April 22 his son-in-law, Dr. Waltman Walters (Phoebe's husband), operated on Dr. Will's stomach. He seemed to rally, and three weeks later Dr. Charlie decided his brother was well enough to be left. Dr. Charlie and Edith traveled to Chicago for a medical meeting. But while in Chicago, he suddenly became ill with pneumonia, just like Dr.

Judd less than four years earlier. It was a virulent form of pneumonia which, in the days before antibiotics, was almost always fatal. Dr. Charlie wanted to fly home to the Clinic for treatment, but his Chicago doctors advised against it. Instead, he was treated at Chicago's Mercy Hospital by five doctors, two of them coming from Mayo Clinic.

When it was evident Dr. Charlie would not recover, Edith called her children and Ruth to come, and they hurried to his bedside. Dr. Will, too weak to travel, had to remain at home.

Dr. Charlie was put under an oxygen tent. Toward the end, he asked that the oxygen be removed so his dying would not be prolonged, and his wish was granted. According to Dr. Chuck, "He looked directly into the eyes of all of us in turn, whispering 'Love' to each. Mother was last; he took her hand and looked at her for a long moment and then weakly said, 'Love.' And closed his eyes. Mother said, after a while, 'This is the way he lived, and this is the way he is dying.'"

He slipped into a coma, and on Friday, May 26, 1939, he died. He was 73.

News of his death immediately went around the world by radio and telegraph. An extra edition of the *Rochester Post-Bulletin* for May 26 devoted the entire first page to the story, a full banner headline across the top reading "Dr. Charles H. Mayo Dies." Their lead news story, after telling details of his last days, gave this tribute: "Rochester's 'Dr. Charlie' is gone, and a stunned city, bowing with grief to time's relentless dictate, paid tribute to a distinguished son who will be remembered both as a surgeon and honored citizen. In this city he spent a life rich in accomplishment and service, and because of his nature, because he was a citizen with a smile and word of cheer for all, and because Rochester's growth was linked indissolubly with him and his famed brother, the memory of him will be a living thing as long as Rochester lives."

The family rode back with Dr. Charlie's body on the train. They were mostly silent, but Edith kept jumping up and leaving the others, to go and stand beside the coffin. That night at home Edith's grown daughters drew lots to decide which of them would sleep with her; they wanted to shield her from the loneliness of life without Charlie. Louise won. She said her mother "seemed like such a little child. 'Dear Charlie! Dear, dear Charlie!' she kept saying."

Throughout the next days, Edith kept her composure. Her son attributed this to her stoic Scots-English family upbringing. The only time he saw her break her poise was when she first saw her husband's body after the undertaker had prepared it for public viewing. She was outraged that he had trimmed Dr. Charlie's luxuriant eyebrows. "She loved the tangle of them," Dr. Chuck said, "and fumed when she found them neatly clipped."

For six hours on Sunday, May 28, Dr. Charlie's open casket, flanked by two honor guards from the Rochester American Legion, lay in state in the 1914 Mayo Building. Appropriately, this building stood on the site of Dr. Charlie's birthplace. Ten thousand people passed his bier to show their respect. His body was then taken to Mayowood. On Monday morning, Dr. Charlie's grandchildren gathered roses into a pony cart and brought them to the house. According to Muff, they were encouraged to scatter them around his body and even behind his ears and in his pockets. "It took away the spirit of death for them," she said.

A funeral service was conducted for family and very close friends at the Big House. For both this service and the public one, Edith dressed herself completely in white, which surprised her family, since she usually wore black.

The coffin was carried along a route in Rochester which included two landmarks: the red house, which Dr. Charlie and Edith had built during the first years of their marriage, and St. Mary's Hospital, where he earned international fame as a surgeon. In front of St. Mary's, hundreds of nurses in their white uniforms, white shoes, and white caps lined the street three deep in hushed silence to show their respect and affection for Dr. Charlie. This sight must have especially touched Edith's heart, reminding her of the days when she was the only trained nurse to work for the Doctors Mayo.

The funeral cortege stopped at Calvary Episcopal Church, where a second funeral service was held. Among the worshippers was Minnesota governor Harold Stassen. The congregation overflowed the small church; three thousand more people stood outside throughout the ceremony. Leaving the church, funeral cars proceeded to Oakwood Cemetery, where Dr. Charlie's body was buried in the Mayo plot. On his gravestone were chiseled the words, "He Lived Abundantly."

The heavy brass doors of the Plummer Building were drawn shut to honor Dr. Charlie; Mayo Clinic closed early, and Rochester businesses closed all afternoon, as a mark of respect. Flowers, telegrams, and letters came from all over the world, what Dr. Chuck called "a weight of mourning that was awesome."

Most of the letters went to the Clinic, but the ones addressed to "Mrs. C.H. Mayo" were delivered to the Big House. Because of the flood of correspondence, Virginia Krause, who had been Dr. Charlie's faithful personal secretary for 13 years, arrived at the Big House each day to help Edith.

Sharing a letter, Edith said, "Oh, Virginia, this is funny. This man is writing to say that 49 years ago, Charlie told him a joke. Afterwards, when they finished laughing, Charlie said to the man, 'Now, don't you feel better? You see – laughter still is the best medicine.'

"The man goes on to say he told the joke over the years a thousand times and always ended it saying 'Now, don't you feel better? You see – laughter still is the best medicine' as if it were part of the joke."

Another letter caused Edith to exclaim "Ohhhh!" and lay her head on her desk, crying. Virginia reached across, put her hand on Edith's shoulder and let her cry. Later she went back to see what that letter said. It was from a woman who wanted to give Mrs. Mayo strength. Her own husband had died that same year, and she only wished that Edith would be strong with that personal and very private loss. It was the only time Virginia saw Edith cry.

Dr. Chuck recalled, "Our grief was personal and, for my mother especially, perpetual. She...carried a miniature of Father's face in her palm always, concealing it in a lace handkerchief. She confided in Alice that it helped her believe that Father was still part of everything she did."

Shortly after the funeral, Edith suggested to Alice and Dr. Chuck that they exchange residences. On June 13, people were moving her furniture to Ivy Cottage while she wrote to Esther. "I still feel like I'm dreaming," she said, "and will awaken and find your Father sitting in his chair by the radio with Peggy on his lap....It is good to be very busy and I'm sure all will be well in the end. I have memories – wonderful memories that will carry me over the top. Soon you will be coming, and Edith – always something to look forward to."

As often as she could, Edith stopped to see Dr. Will. She wrote Esther on July 13, "I stopped to see how Uncle Will has been overnight....He isn't so well. Has never gotten any strength back to speak of, because he has no appetite for one reason. Between you and me, I feel that it won't be many moons before he joins your Father, and I cannot bear to think of both of them leaving us."

Dr. Will continued to lose strength. Dr. Chuck said, "Not long after Father died, Uncle Will noted with professional interest that he was becoming jaundiced. He diagnosed it at once as metastasis in his liver....He reported in a matter-of-fact tone, 'This is it.'"

On Dr. Charlie's birthday, July 19, Edith took some roses to lay on his and Joe's graves. On the way home, she stopped to see Dr. Will. "Found him seeming very small and pale and sweet looking. He wanted to talk about old times – always does when I'm there." On July 22, Edith wrote again to Esther, "Just a line, dear, I have no time to more than say it seems like the world is coming to an end....Uncle Will...is quite reconciled and in [a] cheerful frame of mind. I cannot bear to have anything happen to him. He seems in a sort of way a part of your Father. I'm so sad for Aunt Hattie – the loneliness of it is appalling."

Six days later, Dr. Will died at the age of 78. Dr. Chuck said, "The curious circumstance that the brothers, so bound together in life, should die within two months of one another is something to contemplate. There seemed something natural about Uncle Will's death, once Father had gone."

For Edith these events were momentous. Still, she gradually adjusted to the deaths and was able to continue nurturing her family. The on-goingness of Dr. Charlie's work cheered her. The Mayo Clinic gave the same excellent care to the sick and injured in the days after Dr. Charlie's and Dr. Will's deaths as it had during their lives; the wise and unselfish decisions the brothers had made years before guaranteed no break in quality medical care. Dr. Chuck said, "When my father and Uncle Will died...people speculated on what would happen to the Clinic – nothing happened to the Clinic. It continued without a ripple, thanks to the unselfish arrangements Father and Uncle Will had battled through 20 years before."

In November Edith was able to write Esther, "My dear, don't worry about me. I'm getting myself adjusted to the new way of living....I'm not regretting that I chose to change houses or anything. Of course, nothing could matter of a material nature to make any difference to me, and of course, I'll miss your Father always, just as I do now. I have been so supremely happy for almost fifty years and have only sweet memories of our lives together and at most, it cannot be too long before we are together again....I'd be ashamed not to carry on the best I know how and be thankful for my blessed children than whom no one has sweeter, kinder or more thoughtful."

Named "American Mother for 1940" by the Golden Rule Foundation, Edith traveled to New York City to receive the award, which was publicized in newspapers and magazines across America. To be the winner, Edith had to be judged "the mother representative of the best there is in womanhood." She was declared "a successful mother, as evidenced by the character and achievement of her...children," embodying "those traits most highly regarded in mothers – courage, moral strength, patience, affection, kindness, understanding, and homemaking ability." The Foundation also praised her "for her leadership qualities directed toward aid for underprivileged children and women everywhere." Over the years Edith had served as a leader in establishing Campfire Girls, and she was the first president of Rochester's Civic League. She helped create a Y.W.C.A. in Rochester and even donated her first house, the red house, for its headquarters. Because she understood that wives of doctors studying as Clinic fellows might be lonely, she organized the Magazine Club for them. And for young women employed by the Clinic, 500 of them by 1940, she helped organize the Mayo Clinic Women's Club.

The American Mother award was an event in Edith's family, who came in force to New York to celebrate the honor with her. Dr. Kit Graham, Virginia Krause, Alice and Dr. Chuck, daughter Edith and Dr. Fred with Missey, Ruth, Louise, Esther and Dr. John – all came. Edith was guest of honor at a reception on Friday May 10 and a luncheon the same day at the Waldorf-Astoria Hotel. Saturday she was guest of the New York World's Fair, and on Sunday, Mother's Day, she attended church and then in the afternoon delivered a radio message, broadcast across the nation to millions of people. On Tuesday she was guest of honor at a tea given by the national Y.W.C.A. and a dinner given by the American Mother committee. One New York newpaper correspondent described Edith as "a small slender woman in a simple black dress, her silver hair parted softly above brown eyes that look both wise and kindly humorous." Another called her "a slight, frail woman."

Mrs. Sarah Delano Roosevelt, mother of President Roosevelt, introduced Edith for her radio speech. Edith said she was "deeply grateful" for the honor, but then turned attention away from herself. She called the nation's attention instead to the suffering of innocent mothers and children in Europe, where World War II was already being fought. She asked Americans to place coin boxes on their dinner tables so that "a coin of gratitude would be dropped every time an American family sits down in peace and comfort to partake of an unrationed, bountiful meal." These monies could be sent to relief organizations, Edith suggested.

"I love cards," Edith said, "and I believe in giving

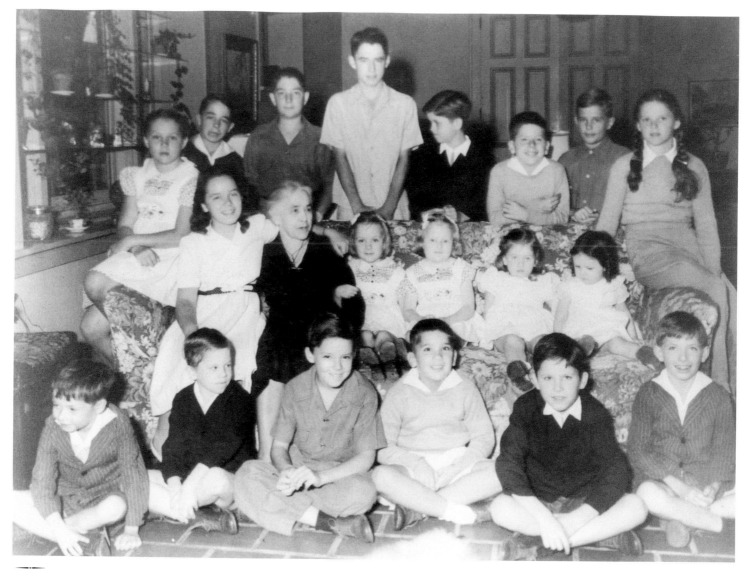

Edith in 1940 with all her grandchildren (Alex Mayo was not yet born)
Top row, from left: Mayo Trenholm (Kooiman), Tom Rankin, George
Trenholm (Elwinger), Fred "Buck" Rankin, Charlie Mayo, David Mayo,
Charles "Bo" Rankin and Mildren "Muff" Mayo. *Middle row, seated on*
coach, from left: Edith "Missey" Rankin, Granny, Prudence
Trenholm, Penelope Trenholm, Ann Mayo Hartzell and Maria Mayo.
Front row, from left: Tom Hartzell, Joe Mayo, Christopher "Kit" Trenholm,
Billy Mayo, Ned Mayo and John Hartzell.

Photo courtesy of Olmsted County Historical Society

cards to loved ones on Mother's Day. But today there
are untold myriads of mothers in Europe and Asia as
well as in impoverished homes of our own land who are
praying not for flowers, but for flour, not for candies,
but for bread, not for greeting cards and telegrams, but
for medicine, sympathy and the necessities of life. If I know
anything about the real heart of motherhood, I do not know
of any way in which we could more appropriately honor
our mothers than by doing for war orphans, widowed
mothers, and victims of military aggression on other
lands, that which we would like to have done for our
own loved ones if conditions were reversed." She
praised the Golden Rule Foundation, "This great
organization is really the 'substitute mother' of millions
of widows and orphans in dire need throughout the
world." Concluding, she said, "Let us all help in this
great work."

A less joyful event of 1940 was the divorce of Louise
Mayo from George Trenholm. Edith had suffered through
the breakdown of that marriage in the late thirties and
the pain it brought her five Trenholm grandchildren.
(Louise later married Leonard Arlin Elwinger.)

Also in 1940, on July 3, Ruth Mayo remarried. She
had met Paul Meserve, a landscape architect from
California, when he was a patient at the Clinic,
recovering from jaundice. Edith and "just home folks"
were invited to the ceremony at 11 a.m. in Rochester's
Congregational Church. Edith described Meserve in a
letter to Esther: he was the same age as Joe, "good
looking – handsome really, fine blue eyes, born and
educated in the East, refined and very likeable." After
the wedding, the couple, along with Ruth's two sons,
lived in the house she and Dr. Joe had shared.
However, Ruth had not fully recovered from her grief
in losing Joe when she married Meserve. He did not
turn out to be what Edith had hoped for Ruth –
"someone with whom you could live happily." The
marriage was stormy with arguments.

Edith had for some time, even before Dr. Charlie's
death, preferred dressing in black. Bo Rankin said, "I
remember her wearing black. Whenever I see her in
my mind, she is always wearing black….To this day, I
think black is a beautiful color."

She continued her habit of prayer. Mayo told of
dropping in to see Granny in the evening, only to find

her busy praying. "'One minute, Mayo,' she'd say. I would sit and wait for her to finish. She was so intent that she would forget I was there. Sometimes I would wait as long as half an hour, when she would turn and say, 'Well, I think that just about covers everyone.'

"She would have Granddaddy's picture (small, in a silver frame, wrapped in a beautiful lace hanky) in her hand. She would wrap it carefully, go to the bed, reach across and carefully tuck it under her pillow…pat the pillow a little and say, 'And that's for you, sweet Charlie.' She would come and give me a kiss and tell me how everyone needed a little help, particularly those who were not within her touch. One time she told me that so many of her friends were dying that when she prayed it was to say goodbye and to help them through the fright and loneliness of death. She did not want them to feel alone."

Bo, too, remembered Granny as a strong Christian. "Granny was the essence of what religion is all about," he said. "She was a role model for all of us—-gentle and humorous, never preachy, even when quoting the Bible and imparting good advice to us. She showed us, not told us, how to live. She was always fun."

Roses took on a special importance for Edith. Dr. Charlie had cultivated flowers, especially roses and chrysanthemums. He had successfully grafted a wild rose onto a domestic rose, creating a lovely hybrid, sweet smelling, with beautiful buds. Edith loved the fragrance of these special flowers. She often wore rose cologne and called it "a gift from Charlie."

On December 7, 1941, the United States entered World War II, and Edith began doing what she could for the war effort. She bought a knitting machine which could knit socks faster than human hands. "It will make me feel I'm still useful," she wrote to Esther. Once a week she and a group of ladies worked at Ivy Cottage, making garments for soldiers. This group became the Zumbro Valley branch of the Red Cross.

One day one of the ladies mentioned a former schoolmate of Edith's, who was sick and alone in the nearby town of Kasson, with no one to care for her. After the women left, Edith went to the phone, dialed St. Mary's Hospital, asked to speak to the nun in charge, told her the sick lady's name, and said, "I want her brought to the hospital right away and cared for. This is Mrs. Charlie. I'll take care of it."

Mrs. Tony, who was German, became more and more aware of rising anti-German sentiment in southeast Minnesota, coming even from the Red Cross ladies. Edith did what she could to protect her. At the sewing sessions, Mrs. Tony said later, "Granny Mayo would never leave my side." After the sewing things were put away, Edith always served tea and cake. She began treating Mrs. Tony with special honor, serving her first at the tea table. After pouring a cup of tea, Edith

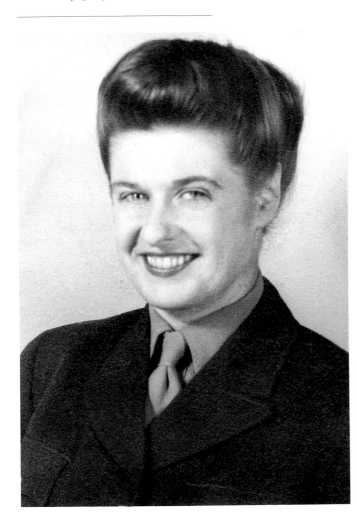

Sally Mayo as a W.A.C.

Photo courtesy of Mayo Kooiman

would ask, "Frau Tony, wunschen Sie Zucker oder Zitrone in Ihrem Tee?" as if German were the most exquisitely polite language in the world. ["Mrs. Tony, do you wish sugar or lemon in your tea?"]

Edith enjoyed playing gin rummy and other games with her grandchildren. George Elwinger would visit his grandmother when he was home on vacation from Breck Military School, and they would play gin rummy "by the hour." He was keen on winning because she paid him in ten cent war stamps when he won. With his winnings, he was able to fill several stamp books and cash them in for war bonds in his name. He said, "I don't remember what my penalty was if I lost; it may have been that I had to play another game."

By this time, Edith's fingers were so clumsy with arthritis she couldn't dress without help, and she had difficulty walking. Nevertheless, Charles Rankin noticed "how easily she managed to be cheerful and genuinely so when she was with her grandchildren."

Calamity shook Edith again in the beginning of 1942. Ruth and Paul Meserve were quarreling often in these days. Then, in the very early morning of February 8, Ruth became violently angry at Paul during a quarrel. She threw her wedding ring from him into the fireplace and ran into their bedroom. Paul followed her in. She pulled open a drawer, grabbed a loaded pistol which had belonged to Joe, and yelled, "If you come near me, I'll kill myself!"

Paul didn't believe her. He advanced towards her to take the gun away; she aimed it at her head and pulled the trigger. A woman guest heard the shot and called Chuck and Alice at the Big House. They rushed to help Ruth, but she died while being transported to the hospital. In shock, Alice and Chuck took the two sleeping boys, David, 11, and Billy, 8, wrapped them in their blankets and carried them home. It was agreed between the couple, almost without words, that they would raise the children with their own.

Dr. Chuck said, "We buried Ruth next to Joe in Oakwood Cemetery. It sickens me that those two passionate and vital people should both have died so brutally, so senselessly, and so soon."

Edith was sickened as well.

⌐◦

Soon afterwards, on April 23, 1942, her last grandchild was born, Alexander Stewart Mayo, son of Alice and Dr. Chuck. She now had twenty living grandchildren, all but seven of them nearby. She found solace in them – playing cards, talking, teaching them through stories.

Several weeks after Alex was born, Dr. Chuck left for Washington, D.C., where he and Dr. James Priestley II trained at Walter Reed Hospital for service in World War II. Eventually, they commanded the two

Dr. Chuck and Edith in late 1942. Edith is wearing the dress in which she would later be buried. Portrait of Joe is on the right, in back.

Photo courtesy of Mayo Kooiman

Mayo Army hospital units in New Guinea and the Philippines.

Late in the summer of 1942, Dr. Chuck returned to Rochester. Edith had been diagnosed at the Clinic with leukemia. She received the news graciously and calmly. From this point throughout the following year of her illness, she intensified her efforts to be useful, especially to her grandchildren. She counseled Mayo to "take the time to find something special to learn or see every day which would create a peaceful feeling inside."

Always a person who lived in the present, Edith redoubled her efforts to see and enjoy. One cold snowy late autumn day, Mayo remembered, Edith invited her to climb up on a windowseat at Ivy Cottage and observe the early morning. Edith said, "What a wondrous day….This makes me feel so young and happy. My eyes witness such fresh glory. Listen to the geese and feel how happy they are to come home to us."

Dr. Chuck and Alice often stopped by the cottage to visit with Edith. They never mentioned her illness, taking the cue from her, despite their distress at seeing a large swelling develop in her neck. Edith always wanted Chuck to talk about the Clinic and his work there. For the first time in her life, she accepted a

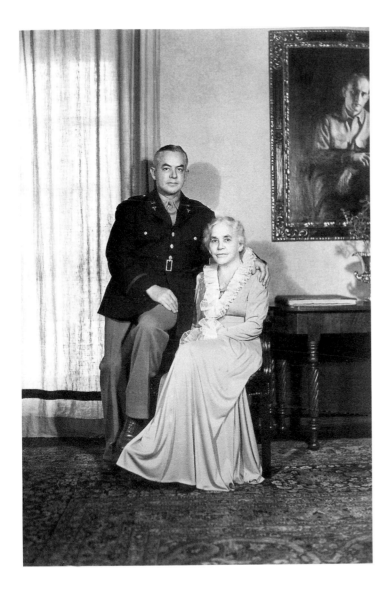

drink during these times with her son, to ease her pain. Chuck would mix her a strong old-fashioned, and they "would talk shop, glasses in hand."

Mayo Clinic shop talk was exciting. Three Mayo doctors – Dr. Walter B. Boothby, Dr. W. Randolph Lovelace, and Dr. Arthur H. Bulbulian – developed, shortly before the war began, an oxygen mask which would enable pilots to fly above 12,000 feet. This mask, named for them the "BLB oxygen mask," was used during World War II in the allied war effort; more than a million masks were produced. In 1942 an acceleration laboratory at the Clinic, with a human centrifuge designed by Mayo scientists, was made available for free use by the U.S. government. Charles Lindbergh was among many distinguished people who visited the laboratory. He made several simulated parachute jumps in the low-pressure chamber in the fall of 1942 and used his research findings in his work developing the P-47 pursuit plane.

Dr. Chuck remained in Rochester until January, 1943. Then he was ordered to Charleston, South Carolina, as director of the Mayo Unit, an affiliate of the 71st General Hospital. His rank was lieutenant colonel. These events Edith followed with interest; like Dr. Charlie, she was intensely patriotic.

During her illness, Edith's physician was her nephew, Dr. John Mayo Berkman (Gertrude Mayo Berkman's son). He decided towards the end that she should be admitted to

St. Mary's Hospital for radium therapy. One day, during Edith's last week, Mayo visited her in the hospital.

"Granny, are you afraid to die?" she asked.

"No," Edith answered. "Aren't we having a good time, you and I? Aren't we warm and cozy here? Aren't we comfortable together, giggling and talking?"

"Yes, Granny," Mayo answered.

Edith continued, "Mayo, you will never forget this warmth between us. Death is such a little thing. All living and loving leads us to this. I will simply get up and leave this room. We will only be a room apart. You are young, and you will never forget me. You may talk to me anytime you need to – I will hear you. I will only be in the next room. You have an entire life ahead of you, but I need Charlie."

Mayo added, "I did not fear for her, for she was so calm, and I feel as an adult that that is what death is – just a room away."

The sisters at St. Mary's Hospital, according to Dr. Chuck, "adored her and fussed over her affectionately." Until near the end, she was conscious and in her right mind. Dr. Chuck said, "She seemed to regard her coming death as a matter of no great importance."

On Monday, July 26, 1943, Edith Maria Graham Mayo died. She was 76. Her family gathered for the funeral. Besides her children and grandchildren, her sister Dinah Graham Olin and brothers Joseph Graham, Jr. and Dr. Kit Graham came.

Edith's body was at first laid out on the antique four poster double bed of carved walnut she had shared with Dr. Charlie at the Big House. The body was dressed in a pale aqua full-length gown with white ruffles, pleated in tiny pleats at the neck and wrists. In her left hand, Dr. Charlie's miniature photograph was placed. Her grandchildren and other close family members came to say their last goodbyes.

Then, her body was placed in a coffin and carried to the sunroom. Each grandchild was given a pink rose to put into the coffin over her chest and hands. Mayo said, "She looked lovely. Then our parents came forward and laid their roses amongst ours. The coffin was closed. I always felt good knowing that Granny was touched by all of us."

Dr. Menefee of Calvary Episcopal Church conducted a private funeral service at Mayowood and another public service at the church, following which Edith's body was buried next to Dr. Charlie's body in Oakwood cemetery. Upon her tombstone, the words "An understanding heart" were written.

In Psalm 91, verse 16, which Edith often heard at church, the Lord promises, "With long life will I satisfy him, and shew him my salvation" (King James Version). After a long life, Edith was satisfied in her passions for healing the sick and for nurturing her family. She was ready to enter the next room.

❋

End Notes

Chapter 1: EARLY LIFE: PIONEERS IN MINNESOTA

Jane Twentyman Graham remembered living in both England and New York state. Her parents, Thomas and Dinah (Chambers) Twentyman, emigrated from Cumberland County, England, to New York state in 1841, when Jane was 13. She left New York state in 1856 at the age of 28, having lived there 15 years.

Chapter 2: NURSING AND PUTTING PEOPLE TO SLEEP

In *Mayo Roots* (published in 1990), page 125, Clark Nelson said Dinah Graham "was the first anesthetist at Saint Mary's Hospital. After her marriage, Edith Maria Graham became anesthetist and trained the Sisters of Saint Francis in nursing at St. Mary's Hospital." This is, I believe, incorrect. It is contradicted in an interview conducted at the Mayo Clinic in 1991, after *Mayo Roots* was published. Edith Olin Batchelder, Dinah's daughter, explained that the sisters began nurses' training together, but illness forced Dinah to withdraw and finish a year after Edith. Dinah was still in school when Edith began working for Dr. W. W. Mayo and when St. Mary's Hospital opened, September 30, 1889. Immediately, Edith organized nursing classes for the nuns, not, as Nelson stated, after Dinah's marriage, which didn't occur until October 31, 1891, two years

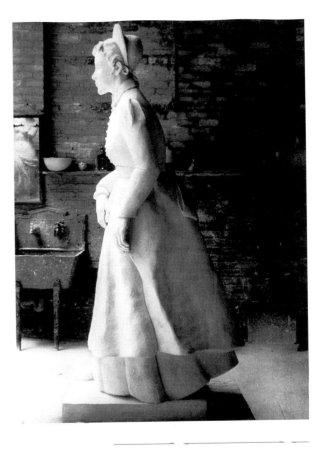

Statue of Edith by artist Mayo Kooiman. The photo was taken in the art studio where it was sculpted by Mayo. In 1953 it was bronzed and presented to St. Mary's Hospital, where it stands in the courtyard, the first statue of a nurse erected in America.

Photo courtesy of Mayo Kooiman

later. While I cannot find it stated exactly when Dr. W.W. Mayo taught Edith to be his anesthetist, she was the first nurse he taught; Dinah was the second.

Chapter 4: MOTHERHOOD

Musetta was the child of Edith's oldest brother, William Beck Graham, and his wife, Grace Frances Morrow Graham.

The Grahams were a healthy, long-lived family. Joseph Graham, the father, lived to be 91, as did his son and namesake, Joseph Graham, Jr. Dr. Christopher Graham lived to be 96. Not including Jennie, the average length of life of the other eleven adult children was 78; Jennie's death at age 25 was seen by the others as grievous and untimely. Her son, Donald Graham Williams, was only two when his mother died. He was adopted by his older aunt, Margaret Graham Twentyman (wife of William Twentyman), who was childless, except for him. Thereafter he was known as Donald Graham Twentyman.

Dr. Millet had died suddenly and untimely——at the age of 39——in 1907 from Bright's disease. Struck blind while on duty at the hospital one day, he died soon after. Dr. E. Starr Judd was hired to replace him, so that the partnership eventually included Dr. Will, Dr. Charlie, Dr. Christopher Graham, Dr. Plummer, Dr.

Judd and Dr. Balfour. In addition to the partners, the permanent diagnostic staff of doctors in 1914 numbered 17, and the clinical assistants 11.

Chapter 6: THE CHILDREN AND THE CLINIC MATURE

"Het up" is slang for "sexually aroused" as well as for "angry."

That Esther Ellis was named for Esther Mayo is a probability, not a certainty. Esther Ellis's cousin, Muriel Melby, wrote me on November 8, 1999, "I cannot honestly say Esther was named for Esther Mayo, but I guess I assumed that she was, as I don't think we have 'Esther' in any of the Stedman, Ellis, or Womelsdorf (Grandma Ellis' family name) families. I have the genealogy for our Ellis line back to 1716….The Womelsdorf line goes back to 1724."

Chapter 7: GRANDMOTHERHOOD

Frances McClure continued caring for Dorothy until June 5, 1960, when an auto accident took Dorothy's life. She was walking across a street in Rochester when a shaft of sunlight momentarily blinded the car driver, who hit her and injured her so seriously, she died an hour later. At her funeral, many people expressed grief. She was deeply loved, especially by the family and by the nuns at St. Mary's Hospital, who knew her well because she had worked for them for many years.

Mayo said of her Aunt Dorothy, "The nuns…were

very considerate of her. A great deal of love was given to her. I was sick when she died."

Chapter 8: THE FINAL YEARS

Muff Mayo wrote me a strong letter contending that Dr. Joe's dog was a golden labrador, not a golden retriever. She even sent pictures of the two breeds, so I could see the difference (which I already knew, but it shows how strongly Muff felt). Dr. Joe liked to duck hunt, she said, and the lab is the right dog for water retrievals. Also, she said that the dog's name was "Fugie." She might be right. But she was only eight when her uncle died, and the written report in Dr. Chuck's book said the dog was "Foosie," and she was a golden retriever. I stayed with Dr. Chuck's description. He was 38 at the time of his brother's death and should have been able to correctly identify the dog.

It was a tough choice for me though. I'm certain that Muff was smart enough at eight to take careful notice of the dog, and is smart enough now to remember her.

Bibliography of Works Used

"America's Castles" presentation on Mayowood. Public Broadcasting System video, 1999.

Batchelder, Christopher. Interview with his mother, Edith Olin Batchelder. In Mayo Clinic archives, "Edith Graham Mayo" file, Summer, 1991.

Beck, Carolyn Stickney, Ph.D. *Teamwork at Mayo: An Experiment in Cooperative Individualism.* Rochester, MN: Mayo Press, 1998.

Brunholzl, Brunhilde. Interview with Judith Hartzell June 14, 1999.

Chapman, J. H., Jr. Letter in Mayo Clinic archives, "Edith Graham Mayo" file, 1887.

Clapesattle, Helen B. *The Doctors Mayo.* Minneapolis, MN: University of Minnesota Press, 1941.

Elwinger, George Trenholm. Undated letter to Judith Hartzell received October 15, 1998.

Hartzell, Dr. John Mayo. Interview with Judith Hartzell, October 10, 1998.
Uncatalogued letters from Edith Graham Mayo et al.

Harwick, Harry J. *Forty-Four Years With the Mayo Clinic: 1908-1952.* Rochester, MN: Mayo Clinic Press, 1957.

Helmholz, Dr. Fred, Jr. Interview with Judith Hartzell, September 16, 1999.

Hodgson, Harriet W. *Rochester, City of the Prairie.* Northridge, CA: Windsor Publications, Inc., 1989.

Kaplan, Anne R. and Marilyn Ziebarth, ed. *Making Minnesota Territory*, 1849-1858. St. Paul, MN: Minnesota Historical Society Press, 1999.

Kirklin, Eleanor Judd. Undated letter to Judith Hartzell, late July, 1999. Phone interview with Judith Hartzell April 18, 2000.

Kooiman, Mayo Trenholm. E-mail letters to Judith Hartzell between October 16, 1998 and June 15, 1999.
Interview with Judith Hartzell September 20, 1999.
Uncatalogued letters from Dr. Christopher Graham to

Edith Graham Mayo.

Life magazine, November 23, 1936, page 19.

Lord, Penelope Trenholm. Uncatalogued collection of letters, newspaper clippings, and photos.

Lowry, Mark. "The Graham Connections" (a genealogy). Rochester, MN: mimeographed by author, 1968.

Mayo, Dr. Charles Horace. Unpublished speech, "Early Days of the Mayo Clinic." Delivered at the Medical History Club, Little Green House, Rochester, MN, February 5, 1929. In George Trenholm Elwinger letters.

Mayo, Dr. Charles Horace II. Interview with Judith Hartzell October 22, 1998.

Mayo, Dr. Charles William. Hand-written *Journal*. In Mayo Clinic archives, 1916.
   Mayo: The Story of My Family and My Career. Garden City, NY: Doubleday, 1968.

Mayo, Edith Graham. "American Mother of the Year Program" speech, May 12, 1940, from Penelope Lord letters.
   My Trip Abroad, unpublished journal of her trip to Europe in June, July, August, 1914. In Hartzell letters.

Mayo, Louise. *Louise Mayo Recollections With Mayo Kooiman*, audio tapes. Interview with Clark W. Nelson at Mayo Clinic, 1976.

Mayo, Mildred. Letter to Judith Hartzell May 5, 1999.

Mayo Clinic, Rochester, MN. Letters in their archives.
   "Mayo History" pamphlet. Rochester, MN: Mayo Press, 1997.

Mayo Clinic, Scottsdale, AZ. "Inside Mayo Clinic," a PBS presentation on videotape, 1992.

Melby, Muriel. Letter to Judith Hartzell November 8, 1999.

Meloney, Mrs. William Brown. "Mrs. Mayo, Wilderness Mother," article in *The Delineator*, September, 1914, pages 9

and 46. From Lord letters.

Nelson, Clark W. *Mayo Roots, Profiling the Origins of Mayo Clinic*. Rochester, MN: Mayo Foundation, 1990.

"Dr. Charlie and the Automobile," article in *The Mayo Alumnus*, page 37.

Olmsted County Historical Society. Letters in uncatalogued boxes and letters in Box R-220.

Rankin, Charles Mayo. Letters to Judith Hartzell October 8 and December 16, 1998, and January 25, 2000 plus undated comments on the first draft of the manuscript, received early May, 1999.

Rankin, Edith Mayo. Audiotape interview conducted by her granddaughter, Karin Rankin Sisk in October, 1978. From Karin R. Sisk private collection.

Redden, Edith Rankin. E-mails to Judith Hartzell March 18 and May 31, 1999.

Rochester Post Bulletin, microfilm collection at O.C.H.S., Rochester, MN.

Walters, Waltman. Interview with Judith Hartzell June 24, 1999.

Warner, George E. and C.M. Foote. *Plat Book of Olmsted County, Minnesota, 1878*. Philadelphia, PA: Warner and Foote publishers, 1878.

Wilcox, Ella Wheeler. *An Erring Woman's Love*. New York City: Lovell, Coryell & Co., 1892.

Wilder, Lucy. *The Mayo Clinic*, second edition. (First edition was 1936.) Springfield, IL: Charles C. Thomas, Publisher, 1955.

Withers, Barbara. Letter to Judith Hartzell August 19, 1999, and phone interview with Judith Hartzell on April 18, 2000.

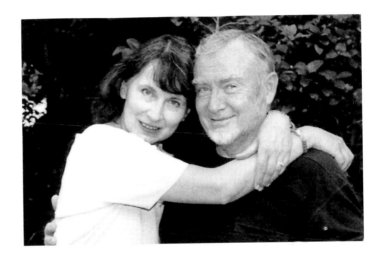

Judith Hartzell with her husband Tom.

Photo by John Berk

Judith Hartzell is a freelance writer who especially enjoys writing and reading biography. She was educated at Cornell University and earned her master's degree in English language and literature from the University of Michigan. Married to Tom Hartzell, Edith Mayo's grandson, she heard stories of this notable lady for many years before beginning to collect them on paper.